MW01517811

THE EMOTIONALLY INTELLIGENT WOMAN

MASTER YOUR EMOTIONS, COMMUNICATE FEARLESSLY AND LEAD WITH CONFIDENCE

THE EMOTIONALLY INTELLIGENT WOMAN

MASTER YOUR EMOTIONS, COMMUNICATE FEARLESSLY AND LEAD WITH CONFIDENCE

DR. SHYAMALA KIRU

To request permissions, contact the publisher at info@lifetopaper.com.

Hardcover: 978-1-777-3736-2-7

Paperback: 978-1-7780111-1-5

Ebook: 978-1-7773736-3-4

First paperback edition February 2022.

Edited by Tabitha Rose & Flor Ana Mireles
Layout by Brady Moller
Photography: Brooke Schall

Printed in the USA.
1 2 3 4 5 6 7 8 9 10

Life to Paper Publishing Inc.
Toronto | Miami

www.lifetopaper.com

To my daughter - you are my heart and my why. My dearest Flamingo, the ideas in this book exist because of you and for you. Thank you for co-creating The Emotionally Intelligent Woman with me - *she exists in each of us.*

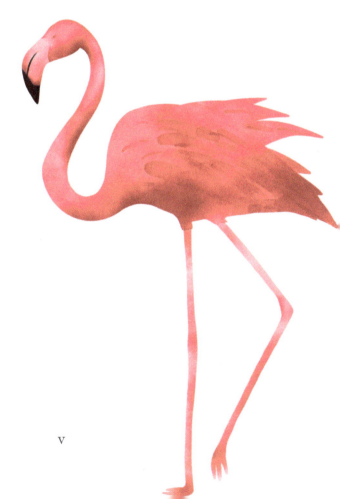

"All Things Change When We Do."
As seen in the waiting room of my first mentor's office.

Author unknown.

Table of Contents

I Took My First Step   1
Honesty Commitment Contract   10

Part One   11
    Master Your Emotions
Chapter one   13
    The Traps Of Our Thinking
Chapter Two   31
    Dig Deep To Get To The Core: YOUR BELIEFS

Part Two   49
    Communicate Fearlessly
Chapter Three   51
    Communication Culprits
Chapter Four   67
    The Assertive Mindset
Chapter Five   77
    There Are Emotional Needs, Then There Are Emotions And Needs
Chapter Six   87
    R.E.A.L Talk
Chapter Seven   103
    Let's Get To The C.A.S.E. - The Assertiveness Framework

Part Three   113
    Lead With Confidence
Chapter Eight   115
    The Toxic Tango Of Relationship Habits

Chapter Nine   131
        Togetherness
Chapter Ten   145
        Separateness
Chapter Eleven   153
        Build Your Blueprint For Emotional Intelligence

Dear Reader   159
Acknowledgments   161
Bibliography   163
Glossary of Terms   165
About The Author   171
About The EQ Code   173

THE EMOTIONALLY INTELLIGENT WOMAN

MASTER YOUR EMOTIONS,
COMMUNICATE FEARLESSLY AND LEAD
WITH CONFIDENCE

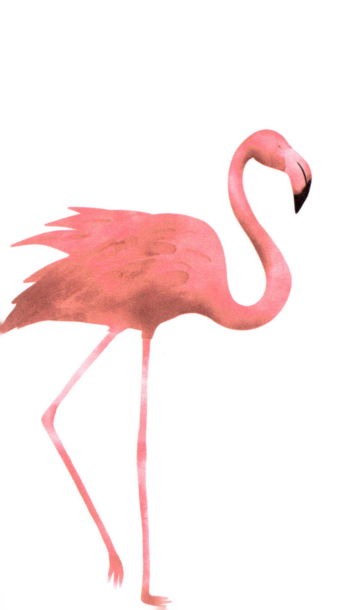

I TOOK MY FIRST STEP

'm out. I can't do this anymore.

The nagging, the bickering and the constant pursuit. The walking out, the shutting down and the cold shoulder. And the worst part? The tension. Followed by never-ending silence. The darkness, aloneness, and fear. I would do anything to never feel that again.

So, I did what any ambitious, high-powered woman would do. I sought help from a therapist. I know what you are thinking, "Wait, were you not the therapist?" Believe me, I was thinking the same thing.

Sitting in the safety of her office, I said, as my eyes filled with tears, "I can't believe I am here; I am a wife, a new mom, and long-time clinician. And most shocking? I am supposed to be a relationship expert. I should know better."

As I wiped my tears, being careful not to smear my mascara, I told her all the things my husband was doing wrong. I told her he wasn't listening to me, "the professional." We were about three sessions in when she said to me, tactfully and gently, you know, that annoying way that therapists do, "It's as if you are throwing a highly sophisticated temper tantrum. Ultimately, you are still behaving like a princess, instead of the queen you are." There it was. My diagnosis: I was an emotionally reactive princess.

Then, it hit me. I was being childish in my relationship, behaving like an emotionally reactive little girl, rather than an Emotionally Intelligent Woman. Having a professional confront me with this reality led to me finally seeing my part in my own story of unhappiness. She allowed me to realize that I was contributing to the tension in my marriage way more than I had ever imagined. I had convinced myself it was all him. For the first time, I realized I had a choice. In fact, I had many choices.

I took the first step and honestly admitted to myself that I had been contributing to the pressure in my home. Though I had admitted it to myself, I still had not admitted it to my husband. My therapist was good, but I wasn't cured overnight. I remember getting the first handwritten receipt for my therapy session, putting it on the kitchen counter for him to see, and not saying a word to him. As I lingered in the kitchen, and slowed down my racing thoughts, somehow, I softened. I don't remember what I said at that moment. What I remember is how I felt when I said it: calm, grounded, responsive. It could have been an innocent question like "Are you ready for dinner?" The content of that conversation does not actually matter. What mattered was that I was no longer saying it in a way that was cold, defensive and full of anxious energy. Suddenly, there was openness, softness and vulnerability. It takes just one person to break the ice and re-route tension. We had dinner. While the room was quiet, it wasn't filled with tension and strained words. Instead, it was filled with the possibility of reconnection. And in the calmness of softer emotions, we saw and heard each other again. Nothing was actually resolved that night. Instead, it began a process of healing, repair and renewed hope.

If you picked up this book, I am going to make a few educated guesses about who you are, at your core. You are an ambitious, high-powered woman. You may even be a recovering type-A, achieve-a-holic who is doing her very best to maximize the life she's given. You may even be a professional woman who wants as much success at home as you've experienced at work. I see you. I get you. I am just like you.

You are fuelled by passion, driven by purpose and fully committed to your mission. You want to be seen, understood, and valued, but you keep getting in your own way. You long for deep, authentic connections, but in your heart, you know that something is missing. You often wonder if there is some sort of secret to better relationships and that next level of success that you have yet to discover. A secret that might make way for the sort of life you have always dreamed of.

You know that your life is meant for more. You also know that you are stuck. What you might not know is that you are being held back by your old beliefs, long ago written narratives and a history of misinformed, unhealthy patterns. You are struggling because, despite how bright, brilliant and beautiful you are, you are your own worst enemy. You are beginning to realize that the ways in which you think, communicate, and navigate your relationships are wreaking havoc on your ability to execute at your fullest and wildest capacity.

That was me, too, over a decade ago. I had just become a mom, started a private practice and signed a contract to appear as an expert on National TV. While everything looked so good on paper, I was struggling more than I ever imagined.

Then, slowly, I surrendered to the idea that I was the only person responsible for my happiness, fulfillment and success. It was mine to own. It was mine to craft. It was mine to create. I finally decided I was out of the blame game. I said goodbye to bitterness, resentment, and wry anger. I said goodbye to loneliness, despair, and self-pity. I was done playing the victim, blaming others and losing myself in the process.

I chose to take empowered action, to take radical responsibility for my happiness and work toward crafting the life and relationships of my dreams. I have a strong sense this is what you want, too: personal power, confidence, elevated relationships, limitless success

The Emotionally Intelligent Woman is a roadmap that is meant to give you the opportunity to create a new paradigm for how you show up in your own life. This roadmap is the one you deserved to have from birth. Together, we'll craft a blueprint that will allow you to hold your personal power in every conversation, every relationship and every context, without fear, guilt or aggression. This book is meant to help you radically improve every aspect of your life. This book offers you a fresh perspective to the old narrative that can leave you feeling lost, confused and stuck in the same old patterns. My hope is that, as you read these pages, and open your heart and mind to what is possible, you will also give yourself permission to be the woman you know you were created to be. Picture these pages as portals, offering you a transformative journey towards your most embodied, radiant and powerful self, crafting the life and the relationships you deserve.

I believe when we have the ability to elevate our Emotional Intelligence (EQ) and our relationships, we are not only able to contribute fully to our mission, but have the ability to show up fully for those who matter most. My mission is to help you unlock the freedom that Emotional Intelligence offers and BECOME the woman who can embody the desires of her heart. For this purpose, I have designed a unique three-part methodology.

Part One of this book is about **Emotional Mastery**. This is the fundamental pillar of success that allows you to manage your emotions, your moods, and your mindset, and take complete responsibility for your own happiness. You will learn how your mind operates, both on a conscious and subconscious level, and how to utilize your mind as the most powerful tool you have. The goal of this section is to equip you with the understanding and strategies required to master your emotions and take control of HOW you respond to others and the world, regardless of what life throws at you.

Part Two of this book is about **Fearless Communication**. Traditionally, women have been taught all the wrong, ineffective ways to communicate their needs. In this section, you will understand the massive difference between toxic communication styles and the fearless communication style. In fact, there is only ONE style of communication that is effective and predictive of better conversations, better relationships and increased confidence. It is time to stop communicating like a little girl and start communicating like an Emotionally Intelligent Woman.

Our final pillar of success is **Part Three: Lead with Confidence**. Here, you will understand what creates tension, distance and decreased intimacy in relationships, which creates a lack of trust within yourself and your loved ones. I will teach you what is needed to navigate your relationships in a way that not only builds your confidence, but also builds better relationships. You will get out of toxic patterns, learn how to be both independent and engaged in your connections, lead with confidence, and uncover why freedom is the best kept secret of relationships that are increasingly stronger over time.

These three pillars of success are what will help you leverage Emotional Intelligence in order to unlock success in every area of your life, accelerate your mission and show up for the people you love.

I believe, at such a profound level, that a lack of skills in Emotional Intelligence is the strongest predictor of overall dissatisfaction in life and decreased success towards our goals. In nearly two decades of practice, I have seen thousands of women struggle to navigate their life and their relationships, and I have seen, first-hand, the impact this has on their confidence, their capacity for contribution and even their mental health.

I was originally trained as a psychotherapist and couple and family therapist, and practiced with passion and gratitude for almost two decades. I am the proud founder and director of the Kiru Psychotherapy Clinic, where I lead an incredible team of dedicated clinicians in the service of innovative mental health solutions for individuals, couples and families.

I am also the proud founder of The EQ Code, a global coaching company dedicated to helping professional women and female entrepreneurs leverage Emotional Intelligence to increase their capacity for success, both personally and professionally. Based on our unique methodology, participants are taken through a transformational step-by-step process that allows them to master their emotions, communicate fearlessly and lead with confidence, so they can execute on their mission at a whole new level.

To say that I love my job is a massive understatement.

In addition, I am a podcast host, media expert for national television, and I have served on the Board of Directors of the Ontario Association for Marriage and Family Therapy. My husband tells me I am slightly obsessed with the intersection between Emotional Intelligence, better relationships and fully embodied leadership. The man is not wrong!

Beneath all the professional accolades, years of service and proud accomplishments, there is really only one reason I found this work. Or perhaps the work found me. You see, when I became a mom, my world completely changed. Motherhood stirred up unresolved issues, a sense of fragility and a never-before-felt sense of inadequacy.

Thankfully, motherhood also stirred up a wild hunger for growth, an insatiable desire for personal expansion and a never-before-felt sense of possibility and determination.

What if it was possible to show up for my daughter as my absolute best self? What if it was possible to lead her as I lead myself? What if I could raise her to become an Emotionally Intelligent Woman so that she could have every opportunity her heart desires?

Then, came the most important question that filled and flooded my heart: WHO would I need to BECOME in order to lead by example at this level?

The Emotionally Intelligent Woman was born after my daughter was born. *The Emotionally Intelligent Woman* emerged from a deep calling to lead myself so that I could lead others, and most importantly, lead my daughter.

While I am proud of all the roles I play, there is one role that is the heartbeat of my mission: Chief Inspiring Officer to my daughter, who I lovingly call "Flamingo." I want to SHOW her what is possible for us. I want her to have a LIVED experience of uncapped potential, self-leadership and personal power.

> *Flamingo, my love, this book was written because of you, for you and with you in my heart, mind and soul. You are the co-creator of these concepts and the co-author of these words. Thank you for calling me to my highest self, and for your love and patience as I get there.*

If you feel deeply called to become your highest self, this book is for you. If you have a purpose burning inside of you and you are ready to give birth to it, this book is for you. If you are prepared to lead yourself in the service of leading others, whether that is personally or professionally, this book is for you.

You are in the right place, and I am so glad you are here.

Are you ready to fundamentally transform the way you think, feel and behave?

Are you ready to unlock personal power and use it to elevate every aspect of your life?

Are you ready to learn to be honest with yourself so that you can be more transparent with others, make mistakes and have the courage and integrity to ask for what you desire?

Are you ready to take radical responsibility for the life that is before you?

Finally, are you ready to lead yourself as you harness the beauty, power and freedom of the Emotionally Intelligent Woman?

I recognize that starting is the hardest part of any journey. If I knew how profound, intense and even painful at times the journey would be, I may never have started. When I started my own journey, I wanted to talk myself out of it. I wanted to press stop, hit delete and move on with my day. However, I didn't, and maybe you shouldn't either. Instead of running away, what if you faced the fear, stayed the course and took the risk of actually transforming your life?

So, here are a few simple things you can do right now to take the next step:

Just start. Don't overthink it, and know that how you start is never how you finish. After all, this is a journey, and we have got a long road ahead of us of personal growth and evolution, over a lifetime.

It is time to face the fear, the insecurity and the inevitable sense of inadequacy that comes with living life out loud, fully and unapologetically. Choose to take the road less traveled and live a life of impact, influence and wild intent.

With that said, my commitment to you is that, I, Dr. Shyamala Kiru, do solemnly swear, that I will:

ϕ Provide you with a proven framework that guides you in your journey of becoming an Emotionally Intelligent Woman.

ϕ Offer you strategies to recognize where your own mindset may be holding you back and how to shift to master your emotions, lead with confidence, and communicate fearlessly in *all* of your relationships.

ϕ Help you achieve those bigger-than-life dreams I know you have.

ϕ Help you adjust your Emotionally Intelligent crown so you can stand tall like the queen that you are.

*As I have committed myself to you, I ask that, now, you commit to **yourself**. Take this seriously. Commit to the most essential part of doing this work, and that is **honesty**. Honesty is your gateway to transforming the way you think, feel and behave. Being completely honest with yourself is the first and most critical step to any transformation. Honesty is going to allow you to learn to let go so that you can fully execute on your mission.*

HONESTY COMMITMENT CONTRACT

I, _____, do solemnly swear to be fully honest and transparent with myself from this moment on.

ɸ I am committed to owning my flaws rather than hiding them.

ɸ I am committed to learning about the parts of myself I think other people may reject.

ɸ I am committed to being honest with myself when it comes to the mistakes made as I embark on this journey of personal expansion and radical change.

ɸ I recognize that being kind to myself during this process means being true to who I am and being honest about where I am at.

ɸ I am dedicated to staying the course and seeing through on this commitment to myself.

_____

Signature & Date

Part One

Master Your Emotions

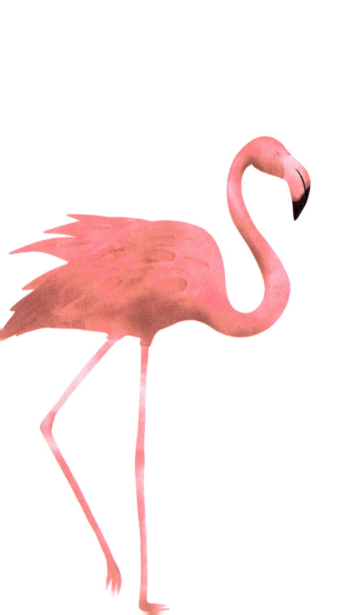

CHAPTER ONE

THE TRAPS OF OUR THINKING

"The problem = your mindset.
The solution = your mindset."

"M ummy, what is wrong?" my daughter asked, interrupting my thoughts from the backseat of the car. Somehow, she *knew*.

I didn't understand how. I had not said anything to indicate how twisted up I was inside from ruminating the night before and being trapped in my thoughts. She couldn't even see my face, but there was no more denying that my little girl could feel it.

I replied quickly, "Nothing!" Exactly what my mother would have said to me in similar situations when I was around four, my daughter's age at the time. That was when I realized she, too, could sense it, just like I had been able to.

I wanted to convince my daughter that she was wrong. I wanted to keep hiding and pretending, even though it wasn't working. I didn't even want to admit that she noticed. I tried to tell myself I was skilled at covering it up, but situations like this would often happen in the mornings when I would drive her to school. I had to pretend everything was alright, hold her little hand and walk her onto the playground, and then proceed to my clinic where I would help other women with their lives and their relationships.

There were so many moments where I would drive over to my clinic feeling like such a failure. I was really struggling, unable to be present with my daughter, and the worst part was that I couldn't admit it myself. I felt like I couldn't tell anybody. I thought it was better to bury it, but when I would get to work and sit in that chair at my office, I knew this wasn't the way I wanted to deal with it. I knew I needed to be honest and work through these difficult emotions, but I just couldn't bring myself to do it. I couldn't bring myself to change. I would think, "What was on my mind that made me react like that? Why was it so hard to manage my emotions when I got stuck in my head?"

I would easily get caught in a well-known mind trap called catastrophizing, thinking the situation was so much bigger than it was. I wouldn't be able to pull myself away from the worry. Then, one day, it hit me: that is what my mother did. I was that little girl so many times, sensing my mother was upset, but unable to verbalize her feelings when I asked her about them. Worse, my mother wasn't able to stop worrying. She didn't have the tools to escape her negative thinking. It was one of the ways her thinking trapped her, and now, the same thing was happening to me, something I swore would never happen. Am I the only one that found myself caught in patterns I promised myself I would avoid at all costs?

YOUR THINKING TRAPS ARE TRAPPING YOU

Your thinking can paralyze you, just like it had done to my mother and had started doing to me. Fear is simply a construct that exists in the landscape of your mind. It isn't real. It might feel real, but I can assure you, it's not.

Here is the good news. The solution is also your thoughts, or more accurately put, your mindset. To master your emotions is essentially to master your mindset. You need to identify your thinking traps, which are what create fear, making it hard to manage anxiety, take risks, and feel confident. Your ability to overcome fear is the difference between a high-powered mindset and one rooted in feelings of anxiety, stress, and overwhelm.

Let me put it this way: we have about 70,000 thoughts per day. If we are unaware and unintentional about our thinking patterns, 80% of these thoughts are negative, and 98% are simply repeated from the previous day. Our mindset, if left unmastered, is geared towards the negative. Essentially, we are repeating old, negative thought patterns consistently, consciously and subconsciously. Developing awareness, adopting a balanced perspective, and taking action despite your negative predictions can free you from your thinking traps. To radically shift the way we think, we must take the 70,000 thoughts that run through our minds each day and look at them as 70,000 opportunities to change and develop a mindset that is optimized for success and growth.

When you operate out of a fear-based reality, you get caught in thinking traps. Getting stuck in a thinking trap is really getting caught in the grips of fear, but I promise you there is a way out.

In two decades of working with people, I have met countless well-intentioned women with the desire to live a mission-fueled life, but who have also felt trapped by one particular issue: fear. Fear becomes so significant that it ends up permeating every part of their lives, seeping into all of their relationships.

Fear is the kryptonite of your mindset. It only exists in the landscape of your mind and often is not reflective of reality. It is crippling, and it is what keeps you stuck, quiet and small. It threatens to consume you with feelings of abandonment, rejection, and isolation. It seals your lips and limits your choices. It traps you in every way imaginable. However, when you do not give into the fear, you can alter your mindset, and in turn, change your entire life.

CATASTROPHIZING:
IT'S ACTUALLY NOT THE END OF THE WORLD
(Even If It Might Feel Like It)

You know those times when you fixate on something so much, where you turn it over and over in your mind, again and again? There are no solutions to be found when you ruminate in these thoughts. There are no new perspectives. There is only increased anxiety. Enter centre stage: Catastrophizing.

Think of catastrophizing as imagining the worst possible outcome AND predicting you will be unable to cope with it. It's twofold, a double whammy, a recipe for immobilizing fear. It's telling yourself, "I am going to fail so badly that everyone will laugh at me AND I will never survive the embarrassment" or taking a relatively small event and imagining the worst possible scenario.

Catastrophizing is telling ourselves we will not survive, even if it's all a figment of our imagination, and we fall into this thinking trap because we are fearful and anxious about the future. In fact, oftentimes, we are terrified of being invited into the unknown. We catastrophize to manage feelings of shame, inadequacy and rejection. It's a protective strategy, but one gone very wrong, as many protective strategies do. Instead of helping, it traps you in the future and keeps you from the present by filling your mind with negative predictions and dysregulated emotions.

When it comes to new opportunities, fear is often there to overtake you and keep you from saying yes. It begins to dictate what you do or don't do and begins running your life, making your decisions and negotiating your relationships. However, with the right tools, you can escape this trap, and luckily for you, I have got a few up my sleeve.

HONE IN ON YOUR AWARENESS

Now, the first step is awareness, and awareness is what will move you towards the solution. When you catastrophize, you remove yourself from reality and are placed into the fear zone. It is important to become aware of these emotions and adopt a realistic perspective that promotes confidence, possibility and action.

If you are always future-focused, pointed firmly in the direction of your life's work and vision without paying much attention to your everyday life, you are probably falling into this trap. It is mission-critical to have a balanced perspective when we are challenging negative thinking. So, what can help you is writing down these catastrophic thoughts and making them concrete. In fact, the mere practice of writing things down is powerful because, when we write things down, it acts as a pause button, interrupting those ruminating and racing thoughts. Once you have your thoughts written down, identify evidence to disprove the conclusions you have drawn from them, which will help you manage your fear. As you consistently practice disproving your negative conclusions or thoughts, you will be able to overcome what has gotten you stuck, and you will see yourself building real, lasting confidence in yourself and your ability to stop catastrophizing and living in fear.

Questions for Self-Reflection:

φ What do you most often worry about or ruminate on?

φ What did you see your parents worrying about as you were growing up?

φ What would be different in your life if you allowed yourself to stop worrying and instead, focused on the possibilities instead?

LABELING:
TREAT YOURSELF HOW OTHERS WISH TO BE TREATED
(Now Read That Again)

The lives of women today are complex.

Take my own life, for example. I am constantly balancing work and family, teaching others how to better manage their relationships, and practicing how to better manage my own. I am a wife, mother, daughter, sister, friend, and entrepreneur all at the same time. We are all multifaceted, but sometimes, it's easy to forget. There have been many moments where I saw myself through the lens of my shortcomings only, and not my strengths. I, too, fall into one of the most common thinking traps that I see high-powered women getting caught in: labeling.

While confidence is something that we all want, and is actually a cornerstone of Emotional Intelligence and a strong predictor of success, we are killing our confidence whenever we begin labeling. In fact, labeling stems from a lack of confidence. It's telling yourself, "I am not good enough," "I am a failure," or "They hate me." You would be amazed at how many high-functioning people speak to themselves in these ways, using extreme and negative labels when they are referring to themselves. They may not say it out loud, but this is the tape playing in their minds.

We all have self-talk and it's not always a bad thing, but when the narrator is nasty and dictating a narrative we have wed, in vain, then I am here to tell you that it's time to divorce the story and marry the truth.

If you are like me, you wouldn't dare speak to anyone else like this. So, why are you smacking these big, ugly labels on yourself? This sort of negative and limiting self-talk often stems from our families of origin. If you were labeled as a child, or witnessed caregivers' labeling themselves, you may tend to label others and yourself negatively, which restricts you from reaching your fullest potential because you are self-sabotaging your self-esteem. You are limiting yourself significantly and causing yourself to have a very narrow definition of self. The more you engage in this thinking trap, the more you create a habitual sense of criticism, not only aimed towards yourself, but towards others, too, limiting how you see yourself and the world.

IDENTIFY AND CHALLENGE YOUR NEGATIVE LABELS

If you find that you see yourself through a very narrow lens, you will want to expand your self-image so that you are able to see yourself as multifaceted rather than as a singular, limiting label and find that sense of confidence you deserve. Identify the labels that you most commonly use for yourself and or others, like 'stupid' or 'incompetent,' and that is the first step to the solution. Next, you want to begin challenging these negative labels by introducing some strengths based labels.

Questions for Self-Reflection:

φ What are you good at?

φ Where do you shine?

φ What qualities do you have that make you special and unique?

PERSONALIZING:
DON'T TAKE THIS PERSONALLY, BUT YOU TAKE THINGS TOO PERSONALLY

"My mother-in-law looks upset. She must be mad at me again."

Does this sound familiar? I have heard this very statement from my clients many times.

If labeling is simplifying or reducing our self-image, then this next thinking trap could be thought of as the opposite. When we personalize, we imagine that we are far more important than we actually are in the lives of others and we make everything about ourselves.

If something just happened that is quite random and you make it about you or you begin to believe that everything that happens around you is a direct reflection of who you are, what people think and what is expected of you, you are falling into the trap of personalizing. This thinking trap is often prompted by fear and a particular sensitivity towards rejection, whether you have a history of feeling rejected or you simply fear it. It's thinking that everything is about you and everything is a negative reflection of you.

Personalizing is fueled by self-blame, meaning you constantly blame yourself for anything and everything that happens around you, which leads to assuming inappropriate responsibility for things or events that have nothing to do with you. For instance, let's imagine you are about to throw an outdoor party, a barbecue, and out of nowhere, the forecast predicts rain. If you were to personalize that, you might say something like, "Terrible things always happen to me" or "It's always when I decide that I am going to put myself out there that I get shut down." When you personalize things that have nothing to do with you, like the weather, it leads to an unhealthy emotional response.

Let me give you another example.

If my husband has a challenging day at work, it has absolutely nothing to do with me, but if I fall into the trap of personalizing, I can easily make his bad day, and the mood associated with a rough day at work, about me and in fact, make his day worse. This type of thinking leads to often feeling upset because you react to events as if you are personally responsible for them. It leads to emotional breakdowns, increased sensitivity with direct communication, and difficulty having honest conversations, and once you have reached this point, it becomes almost impossible to communicate confidently.

If you cannot communicate fearlessly and have honest conversations, it becomes practically impossible to build authentic connections in your life, which kills your overall confidence, further feeding into other thinking traps. If you are highly sensitive to direct communication and have difficulty having honest conversations, this becomes highly problematic in deepening intimacy, and this lack of intimacy creates an incredible amount of distance or conflict in a relationship, and it can keep you feeling alone and isolated.

BE RESPONSIVE, NOT REACTIVE

Personalizing is one of the most common thinking traps that I see with women, and like most strategies, the key is perspective.

It's not all about me. It's not all about you.

The goal is to remove yourself from the center of the universe and think objectively. The goal is to be responsive, not reactive.

To overcome the trap of personalizing, you must think objectively and begin asking yourself some crucial questions. You need to force yourself to expand your thinking, expand your vision, expand your perspective, and consider all factors because it is highly problematic when you have a very narrow perspective. You need to expand your view and ask yourself, "Am I taking things personally that are not within my control?"

Let's go back to the example of the barbecue that got rained out. Am I telling myself that no one came to my barbecue because nobody likes me rather than acknowledging the fact that it rained and the barbecue was outside? We must ask ourselves what other reasons may account for the way people around us are responding. This is critical because personalizing keeps you stuck and, if you are anything like the thousands of women I have worked with, you do it way more than you might realize.

In order for this healthier mindset to become normative, you will need to work through these questions. Oftentimes, we have blind spots when it comes to how we behave around other people, but if there is somebody in your life that you trust and knows you well, sit down and do this work with them. It will help you gain an alternative perspective, an outside perspective, and help you deepen this whole exercise.

Questions for Self-Reflection

φ *When and with whom are you most prone to taking things personally?*

φ *What insecurities do these personalizations point to?*

φ *What would happen if instead of projecting your insecurities on others, you began working on building your sense of self confidence?*

PERFECTIONISM: IT'S NOT ALL ABOUT YOU

Personalizing and labeling are related to our sense of self confidence. We are in the habit of thinking too little or too much of ourselves. The next common thinking trap, perfectionism, is more about expecting too much of ourselves. It's not a direct reflection of our own confidence, but a trap that sets us up for disappointment in ourselves.

Perfectionism is pervasive in our culture, particularly persistent with women. It hurts us and makes us believe we need to be at 100% capacity 100% of the time. I remember thinking, in order to keep my husband's love, I needed to be the perfect wife, mother, and even professional. With perfectionism, there is no room to fail, and this is highly problematic. It's a real epidemic, and it's something that we need to manage. Now, the only way to manage it is to be intentional with our thoughts.

Similar to our other thinking traps, perfectionism is driven by anxiety and a need for control, and can often lead to burnout. Burnout is often fueled by high-levels of anxiety, perfectionism, and a need for control. It is driven by a fear of inadequacy and rejection and it sets us up for failure. When we say to ourselves, "Listen, I need to get things right 100% of the time," while knowing it's impossible, we allow ourselves to fall into procrastination and reduce our ability to take risks because risks mean that there is the possibility of getting it wrong. Perfectionism does not allow for a possibility of failure, but it goes even deeper than that. It decreases your confidence because you never test your limits to see what you can achieve. It limits your growth because you don't try new things, preventing you from trying and doing something you might enjoy.

PROGRESS > PERFECTION: JUST BE YOURSELF

Now, to overcome perfectionism, you want to begin to identify more realistic standards for yourself and remember that progress is ALWAYS better than perfection. In fact, it's healthier. When I started to record and produce my first digital course for my flagship coaching program, I had this idea that I couldn't fumble or take a breath. I couldn't just be myself even though my clients were telling me again and again that one of the things that they loved about working with me was that I was a real human, flaws and all.

However, now I know, when you are truly yourself and you fully lean into any process, you make it easier for others to connect and relate to you. Nobody wants perfection. Nobody wants that fake, polished image that you see all over social media. Our culture is oversaturated with that. I believe that, more than ever, people are looking for authentic humans, real connections and unfiltered lives.

When you begin to change the narrative of perfectionism and allow yourself to connect with and identify a more realistic standard for yourself, you stop procrastinating and start taking action, and this is exactly what happened for me with my first course; once I let go of the need to get it perfect. I was able to move forward and finish this very important project. Not only did I finish it, but finally telling perfectionism to take a hike allowed me to create several more courses and eventually an entire curriculum for women who want to dial in their Emotional Intelligence. Letting go of perfectionism gave me the key to unlock far more than what I had imagined I was capable of.

When we set more realistic standards for ourselves, we are then able to make room for mistakes, which are not only okay, but actually the pathway for success. We need to embrace failure as the pathway to success because mistakes are truly the way that we live fully and authentically. And I am totally here for it. What about you?

FROM BLACK AND WHITE TO TECHNICOLOR

Have you seen the classic film, The Wizard of Oz? I have seen it dozens of times. Every time I watch it, I feel the magic when Dorothy opens the door to the farmhouse and her world transforms from black and white to Technicolor. It's a moment that always leaves me with a sense of wonder, and this is exactly how I feel about helping women step out of black and white thinking and expand their perspectives.

Black and white thinking is similar to perfectionism, and both could be blamed for the thought, "If you are not first, you are last." Another example of black and white thinking is something I hear a lot of women say: "So, I was supposed to start my diet today, but I have already indulged in chocolate, so now my entire diet and all my health goals are ruined, just like that." This is the epitome of black and white thinking, and it happens when you look at situations in terms of extremes and miss the nuances. It's this inability to hold a balanced perspective and see life in terms of many shades and many hues.

Black and white thinking develops from a fixed mindset, and a fixed mindset does not allow room for growth. It's driven by a fear of uncertainty and a fear of losing control, and creates a very rigid communication style. When you engage in black and white thinking, you are unable to see life and events as a continuum with multiple possibilities and perspectives. This makes resolving conflict in relationships extremely tough because a lack of mental flexibility keeps you from seeing whatever you are arguing about from a different point of view.

Now, this is something I really struggled with early on in my marriage. "Leave me alone," my husband would say to me after hours of arguing in circles. In his mind, it was a disagreement and he needed a break. In my mind, he was done with me and it was time to call divorce lawyers. Dramatic, I know, but this is how it actually played out in my mind.

I hated the sound of those words. They pierced me and sent me into a downward spiral, especially back then when our relationship was still taking shape and the space between us could feel wildly fragile. Each time an argument culminated in those three triggering words, I heard, "Leave me alone, forever. It's over." Meanwhile, what he meant was "Leave me alone for a moment. I need to collect myself, regroup, and come back to you with calmness and clarity."

This gap in our perspective shaped many painful arguments in those early years of marriage for us. I grew up believing that disagreements were never okay, conflict was bad, and that differences in perspective were scary. Meanwhile, my husband grew up believing that opinions are to be expressed, conflict is healthy, and that different perspectives are normal.

We have been together for almost 15 years and we still have disagreements. We still have differences. But as we have made space for both disagreements and differences, the space between us no longer feels so fragile. It feels safe and intimate, and I am grateful that I have learned how to redefine my understanding of what it means to build real intimacy. Now I know it has nothing to do with how much we 'get along or agree on everything,' but about having the courage and integrity to show up when we don't.

BRIGHTEN YOUR COLORS AND BROADEN YOUR PERSPECTIVE

To move away from the insanity that is black and white thinking you must first broaden your perspective. You must make room for multiple perspectives, and understand that the perspective that you are holding is just one perspective, and it is *your* perspective instead of the truth of the situation. You must identify multiple aspects of the particular event, not just the negative aspects. You must put yourself in a position where you are beginning to identify those different shades and nuances that do exist within that continuum and you have got to take the emotion out of it.

Questions for Self-Reflection:

φ Am I seeing this situation with only one or two possible solutions?

φ Am I missing any information?

φ What other perspectives or possibilities exist?

PLAN YOUR ESCAPE

The success of our relationships depends so much on our own mindset. What we bring to the table impacts everything else. It's so important for us to first acknowledge that, by nature, our mindset is negative and repetitive. We remember five unhappy thoughts for every happy one and we think about the same things over and over again each day. These behaviors that once protected us are now responsible for keeping us trapped in our own thoughts, overwhelming us with feelings of fear and anxiety until we become paralyzed.

My goal is to help you radically shift the way you think, feel and behave so that you can find happiness and fulfillment in your life and your relationships. I want to help you realize that this fear isn't real, your thoughts are not always an accurate reflection of your reality, and all you need to do to escape these traps is to change your thinking patterns.

The first step to overcoming this negative thinking is to simply be aware of it. If you find that you are catastrophizing, then write it down and you will likely see clearly how unrealistic these imagined outcomes really are. You can then begin to look at these thoughts critically, unpack them, and begin to let go of the fears that come with them.

When you forget that you are a complex, multifaceted human being and fall victim to labeling yourself, remember to take some time to reflect on what labels you use on yourself most regularly, write them down and pay attention to your mind the next time it tries to use that label. Trust me, you will see that you can't be summed up in one word and you will be able to stop trusting those labels, find confidence in yourself, let go of your ego and stop taking responsibility for every bad thing that happens in your life. you will remember that, sometimes, it just rains, and no one is perfect. So, give yourself a break, explore, try new things, and make the mistakes that are so important to your growth. Remember, ***you are responsible for your own happiness***. By getting really concrete on managing your thoughts, you can master your emotions and build your confidence.

When I look back now on that car ride with my daughter, I am much kinder to myself than I was at the time. I no longer label myself as a failure for having struggles with my emotions and relationships. I no longer expect myself to be the perfect mother. Instead, I acknowledge that I am simply a person doing the best I can with the tools I have and that, despite my own expertise in relationships, I am still bound to make mistakes. I see now how easy it is for a negative mindset to take control. I was lost in my own thoughts. I can't even recall what it was that was on my mind that morning, but I was definitely caught in the trap of catastrophizing.

Worry and fear were habits I chose. I realize now that I can make a different choice. From moment to moment, I can choose faith over fear and courage over worry. In the past, if I was really stressed, it was challenging for me to be fully present and engaged, and that is exactly how I experienced my own mom. The stresses were different, of course, but it didn't really matter because the external circumstances are never the real problem.

My daughter saying, "Mummy, what is wrong" was a transformative moment for me. It wasn't until I started managing situations like that differently, that I realized how poorly I was actually handling them. I needed to become conscious of my own limitations and, more importantly, to the possibilities for change. Now when I wake up, I consciously tell myself to be here, to be present.

Recently, my daughter woke up from a bad dream and wanted a hug from me. The whole experience was different because *I was different*. If this had been in the past, I would have been so focused on whatever stress was going on that I wouldn't actually be there, but that morning, our interaction was different. I actually *felt* her little body, her little back like angel wings, and my voice and touch were offered to comfort and soothe her. It was what she needed at that moment, and it was what I needed. My daughter saying "Mummy, what is wrong" was the turning point I needed to show up for her and for me.

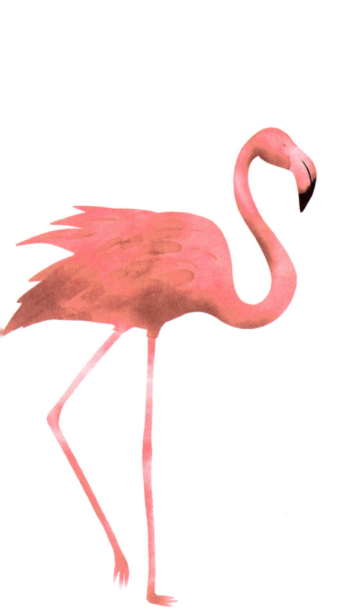

CHAPTER TWO

DIG DEEP TO GET TO THE CORE: YOUR BELIEFS

"Believe you are the master of your mind and your mindset is mastered."

"**W**ho am I to lead at this next level?"

"Am I cut out to do this?"

"Have I somehow slipped through the cracks?"

These may be some of the silent questions you have asked yourself. Maybe, you have experienced this sentiment where you don't feel that you *can* be the person you are wanting to be. If you are playing all in, imposter syndrome is there to greet you. In fact, it's a normative experience for high-powered women, and it can occur at different stages of your career, especially when you are moving from one level to the next.

Over a decade ago, I was hired to be an on air expert on a TV show. I had no prior experience with television, and honestly, the first few seasons were completely cringe-worthy for me. It all felt so strange. I really didn't know how to show up as this confident woman, let alone an "expert." I was stiff and I wouldn't even smile. At every single level of growth, I had felt like an imposter, and right before I would level up, I would feel imposter syndrome coming on, and then, it would hit. I would ask myself, "Who am I to say I am an expert?"

I could never wrap my head around how this was happening to me. A television show needed an on-air therapist, and one of my colleagues recommended me to the producer. So, I auditioned, thinking nothing would come of it, and then, as fate would have it, they hired me. I had felt so out of place and exposed. I was the only female, a petite 4'9 woman of colour, on a panel of all male experts. The crew literally had to put riser cushions on my seat just so that I could be at eye level with the other experts when we were filming. I remember so vividly, in that moment, feeling that deep sense of inadequacy, and that, soon, everyone would catch on to my shortcomings (no pun intended) and the fact that I did not belong in that studio. It went so far as me telling myself I had nothing valuable to contribute and "Who was I to call myself an expert?" For the first five years that I appeared on this television show, I felt forms of imposter syndrome creeping in at various times. Your read that right—imposter syndrome showed up for me for five years straight.

At first, it was scary for me to show up authentically because I had this limiting belief that I wasn't good enough to be on the show. One of the narratives I would say to myself all the time was that I had slipped through the cracks. This was my classic limiting belief about myself: I had definitely slipped through the cracks. They had made a mistake, I slipped in, and eventually, they were going to figure out that hiring me was a mistake. Every year when they asked me back, I was shocked. It didn't matter how many accolades I got or how much positive feedback was offered, I still felt like I didn't belong on television. I remember so vividly after my first day on set, the owner of the production company pulled me aside to tell me I was great on camera and asked me to audition for another show. However, at the time, all I could think to myself was he was making a mistake. I remember questioning what gave him this impression of competence. It didn't matter how many people told me they liked my work on the show, I was convinced I had no business being there. I was flooded with limiting beliefs. Despite having those thoughts, I kept showing up each season, and it was so hard. I would be excited, yet scared, and I could never sleep the night before the beginning of every season.

Needing to show up for this TV show, launching my own practice, being a mom and engaging in my own therapy were all happening for me at a parallel time, and it was becoming exhausting to have to be a different person at work than at home. I felt that I wasn't being true to who I was and who I could be. While I was receiving all this praise, inside, I felt that I was just putting on a facade. I thought I didn't *belong* in the spotlight, and there was something about the cameras that intensified this feeling. I vividly remember thinking that the cameras were going to be able to see through this fake version of myself that I was putting on. That one camera was going to catch my lack of confidence.

It was in this moment that I realized that my life deserved the fullest version of me. *The experience of showing up on camera taught me to truly show up for myself.* What began as one of the scariest things I have ever done, ended as one of the most transformative decisions I ever made.

I stayed on for 10 years. Therapists came and went, but I stayed on until the very last season of the show. It was a defining moment for me that helped me to step into my power, and this experience showed me how important it was to show up fully, as myself and for myself.

Now, I tell you the same thing.

Believe you are the master of your mind and your mindset is mastered. Perhaps you are not on a television show at this point, but you owe it to yourself to show up for yourself. Your life deserves the fullest version of you, cameras or no cameras.

I feel like the first half of my career was identifying the problem, and the second half was working on the blueprint to the solution. What I was noticing was that there was this common thread that ran through every woman I worked with. This fraud-like feeling was in their stories just as much as it was in mine.

I was able to overcome imposter syndrome by really digging deep into the heart of my own mindset by uncovering my core beliefs and what I wanted to achieve for myself.

I needed to determine who I wanted to BE and show up as her. I needed to believe that I was the master of my own life and my mindset.

DEFINING THE VOICE THAT SAYS YOU CAN'T DO IT:
Limiting Core Beliefs

A limiting core belief I had was that I wasn't good enough. Eventually, I was able to overcome it, but I remain vigilant to its demise. This belief is very common for women, and it can get triggered at any point in time, whether in their personal lives or within their career.

Core beliefs... What are they? Well, they are longstanding, enduring beliefs about ourselves, people, and the world. They are those "all or nothing" statements that we make time and time again that tend to have an absolute nature to them, generally on a global scale. These beliefs are what we tell ourselves reality is made up of, despite any evidence that might contradict them. These beliefs inform the way we understand and make meaning of the world around us and our place within it. Because of this, core beliefs tend to have a tremendous impact on our emotional health, and in particular, our self-esteem. Core beliefs can dictate how we conduct ourselves in relationships, and in life overall. This is why it is so important to dig deep and get to the core of what you want for yourself and determine what you want your core beliefs to be.

Regardless of whether they are limiting or not, a question you may be asking yourself is, "Where do these core beliefs come from?" Many of our core beliefs were actually birthed and raised alongside us. They were the unspoken, unwritten rules that our families lived by, and they are the ways in which we move through our relationships and our sense of self based on early childhood experiences. They are definitive in their nature, and if left unchecked, can become our greatest stumbling blocks. As we get older, the goal is to reassess some of these old belief systems and develop new and more adaptive ones.

Ask yourself what core beliefs you hold. Which beliefs are limiting and which beliefs are expansive? Which core beliefs hurt your growth and which ones support your growth? If your core beliefs are adaptive and healthy, then keep them, but if they are maladaptive and unhealthy, then it is important to challenge these beliefs, show up for yourself and reach your greatest potential. In other words, you need to take your limiting core beliefs and transform them into high-powered beliefs.

Questions for Self-Reflection:

φ What are my core beliefs?

φ What core beliefs are limiting me?

φ What core beliefs are helping me grow and become the best version of myself?

HIGH-POWERED BELIEFS = HIGH-POWERED MINDSET

High-powered beliefs are part of a high-powered mindset you can develop, which allows you to live life fully. For me, this is what Emotional Mastery is all about. So, in order to optimize your mindset for your high-powered goals, it is absolutely critical that you dial into your core beliefs and look at the change you wish to create for yourself.

In order to achieve this shift in mindset, you need to begin with small changes, day-in and day-out. When you think about creating change, it is far more effective to practice new positive core beliefs than it is to constantly challenge negative ones. Essentially, what you want to be able to do is identify new core beliefs that you want to hold onto and look for ways to support and strengthen them. This offers you the possibility of taking on a fresh perspective and you can find evidence to support these new core beliefs, which will help you to embed these into your mindset.

Now, you don't need to get rid of negative core beliefs altogether, but what you really want to do is simply disrupt them by introducing more high-powered beliefs.

You may be asking yourself, "What are some of the characteristics of a high-powered mindset? How do I really drill down and identify these characteristics that I want to foster?" Here is the key: small changes, made with consistency, always lead to bigger changes, and eventually high-powered beliefs. So, the first characteristic I recommend is flexible thinking.

LET'S GET PHYSICAL FLEXIBLE

When it comes to high-powered beliefs, it is a matter of mindset and flexibility. The more you can become flexible in your thinking, the more you allow yourself to move away from rigid, negative thinking patterns. What this means is, instead of insisting on a certain outcome or achieving a particular goal, you *prefer* a particular outcome or wish to achieve a certain goal, but you are flexible to the idea of not attaining it. This also means you are able to make room for normal human error and random life events, and become more accepting of alternative outcomes to ones that you were very insistent on having.

Questions for Self-Reflection:

ϕ What beliefs do I hold that are very rigid and limiting?

ϕ What beliefs can I introduce that will allow me to be more flexible in my thinking patterns?

LET'S GET ~~PHYSICAL~~ SENSIBLE

The second characteristic of a high-powered mindset is to be sensible with your thoughts and beliefs. In other words, rather than thinking extremely negative things about yourself, others, or the world based on a single event, try to maintain a sensible and healthy perspective about the event. This is the importance of having a balanced perspective where you approach your negative thoughts with sensibility and remind yourself that no one is perfect, and people are fallible. So, instead of failing at something and viewing yourself as a complete failure, what you want to do is accept the defeat and understand you tried your best. You may be disappointed in yourself for having failed, but it's not the end of the world and you can try again.

Questions for Self-Reflection:

ϕ How can I reframe failure so that it does not defeat me?

ϕ What can I learn from my mistakes and my failures?

KNOW IT'S POSSIBLE

The final characteristic you want to achieve is knowing and understanding that high-powered beliefs and a high-powered mindset are, in fact, possible, and this one is so important. One of the key components to adapting your mindset and digging deep into the core of your beliefs is knowing that it's possible and *real* to challenge your negative thoughts and slowly combat them with positive ones. It's allowing space for the possibility of good, less good, neutral *and* bad elements. It's allowing flexibility *and* sensibility into your life, beliefs and mindset. The world is complex. *You* are complex. Therefore, you want to adopt the perspective that there can be both bad *and* good. It's really about being realistic and honest with yourself while being able to embrace that flexible, sensible, and sometimes nuanced mindset that you have. This is critical for Emotional Mastery.

Questions for Self-Reflection:

φ What high-powered beliefs can I start adopting?

φ What am I working towards achieving in my life right now?

φ What difference would it make if I was able to adopt some high-powered beliefs?

AUDITING YOUR CORE BELIEFS

Now, from time to time, it is necessary for you to audit your core beliefs, and what this means is to get really concrete and take a look at your core beliefs. Now, I have three different audits to share with you to help you achieve this. Refer to and use the following Core Belief Audits as often as you would like to increase your self awareness and take action toward Emotional Mastery.

AUDIT #1: SELF-REFLECTION

Have you ever asked yourself about the decisions you make and how you negotiate your life and your relationships? Do you optimize the power of your mind through supportive beliefs?

The Self-Reflection Audit is an opportunity for you to increase your personal power by increasing your ability to reflect on your own choices. In particular, you will want to identify what is working for you and what is hurting you. It's amazing what can happen when you actually identify these beliefs and increase your awareness around the impact these beliefs have on your day-to-day functioning.

Identify the core beliefs that are hindering your growth. Identify the core beliefs that feel supportive, expansive and allow you to become the woman you desire to be.

Questions for Self-Reflection:

- φ *Which of my choices are hindering my growth?*
- φ *Which of my choices are helping me further my growth?*

AUDIT #2: SELF-AWARENESS + STRESS

The next audit is what I like to call the self-awareness audit.

If you are struggling with self-awareness, or have people in your life that are close to you reflecting on an experience with you and it does not resonate at all, it's much more important to engage with this audit. Self-awareness is absolutely critical to your Emotional Intelligence. In fact, it's a cornerstone, and the goal here is to increase your emotional regulation through self-awareness. This is because, unless you are self-aware, you are unable to regulate your emotions, and this is the biggest block to developing a resilient mindset. Self-awareness is what allows you to manage your emotions and increases your emotional regulation skills, which further allows you to communicate clearly and congruently with all the people you have relationships with.

You may be asking yourself, "How can I increase my self-awareness?" Well, there are certain questions you can ask yourself, like "Do I feel tension in my chest? Do I feel stress in my body?"

To answer these questions, do a self-rating, which can be done on a scale of zero to 10, where zero is that you experience absolutely no stress and 10 is that you experience insurmountable stress.

Questions for Self-Awareness:

1. What is your current level of stress?
2. What is your general ability to cope with stress?
3. What choices do you make when you are stressed?
4. How much does your stress affect your relationships?
5. How much would you benefit by learning to manage your stress?

Low-level stressors are common normal, and these are your 1 to 3, or even 4 self-rating responses. However, if you are constantly rating your stress at a 5, this is something to be aware of and look at. If you are constantly rating your stress above a 5, you may want to make a change in your life and maybe even seek support.

Questions for Self-Reflection:

φ *How self-aware am I of my actions and thinking patterns?*

φ *How is stress affecting my life and the choices I make?*

AUDIT #3: FEEDBACK IS THE FOUNDATION

Feedback is critical to developing a high-powered mindset, and it is critical to your communication style, as well as to building authentic connections. For me, feedback is the foundation for elevated relationships and leading with confidence. We need it, and we need to welcome it. We need to learn to manage our own emotions around feedback, especially when we are anxious to receive it.

The truth is, you probably don't like receiving feedback, and you may even react to it with defensiveness. Perhaps, you respond with defensiveness in your head, but don't communicate it with others directly, or you are visibly and verbally aggressive to others when they give you their feedback. Whatever the case is, feedback is absolutely critical, and it is a critical component of Emotional Mastery and the entire Emotional Intelligence framework for high-powered women. Seeking feedback is an important element of Emotional Intelligence, and you need feedback to develop your emotional and mental resilience, which, in turn, will allow you to communicate fearlessly and lead with confidence. Once you accept feedback, you allow yourself to receive concrete data as to how others perceive you.

The truth is that our perception of how we communicate and come across to others is often inaccurate. Unless you increase your self-awareness and ask for consistent feedback, you are going to struggle with your emotions and, ultimately, your relationships.

The goal of this audit is to improve your relationships by simply getting direct feedback.

Ask the following questions to your family and coworkers:

1. Do you think I get stressed or anxious easily?
2. What do you think is hindering my growth?
3. How do you feel about our relationship?
4. Can you turn to me for help?
5. Do you feel supported and encouraged by me?

Encourage them to be honest with you.

Once your family and coworkers have answered these questions, this is where the magic happens. What you want to do next is debrief the responses *together*. This is powerful because it opens up the relationships you have with these individuals and invites you to get comfortable with the discomfort of receiving feedback. As far as I am concerned, getting comfortable with receiving feedback is a life skill. In addition, it provides an opportunity to form a deeper, more authentic connection with the individuals already in your life. Ultimately, this will allow you to really engage in a conversation about how to improve your relationships, which will be crucial for your Emotional Mastery.

Questions for Self-Reflection:

⚵ *What areas do I need to change or improve in order to grow?*

⚵ *How do I feel about the relationship I have with myself and with others?*

OPTIMIZING HIGH-POWERED BELIEFS

If we are truly going to master our emotions, we need to be creative in our thinking and make space for new optimized high-powered beliefs. This means functioning at our best so that we can not only manage our own moods, but really show up for all the people in our lives that are important to us.

It's an opportunity to step out into uncharted territory and create something new and utterly amazing, not just for yourself, but for your loved ones, too. The goal here is to claim your stakes in the world and live your mission from a place of courage and confidence.

You may ask yourself, "How do I get to this place? How do I arrive at this mindset?" Well, I have got some guidelines for you that will help you optimize your high-powered beliefs. Together, we are going to look at how to develop and hone these mindset muscles, because, just like real muscles, these beliefs need to be trained and worked on if we actually want to master our emotions.

So, what are the guidelines? What are some of the key components to have in your toolbox that you can continue to use for reference as you grow into an Emotionally Intelligent Woman. A high-powered mindset has a few elements that I really want to highlight.

BE TRUE TO YOURSELF AND TO YOUR REALITY

To start, a high-powered mindset is true and consistent with reality. It is *based* in reality and *in touch* with reality, which prevents a distortion or denial of the facts of a given situation or experience. When your mindset isn't consistent with your reality, the truth is, your anxiety goes up and you feel overwhelmed and your emotions become dysregulated. Essentially, you put yourself in a place where your mind is existing in a landscape that isn't in touch and consistent with its surroundings. In these moments, it's really important to identify the thinking traps you fall into and challenge them. It's important to realize the thinking patterns you are experiencing that continue to pull you from the high-powered mindset you want to achieve.

Questions for Self-Reflection:

φ Which of my beliefs position me for growth?

φ Which of my beliefs limit my growth?

ACCEPT THE UNCERTAINTY AND
LEAVE ROOM FOR ERROR

The second guideline to optimizing your high-powered mindset is cognitive flexibility. A high-powered mindset is a flexible mindset. It leaves room for error and allows you to recognize the fallibility of people and that we are all capable of both success *and* failure with any given task. It's the ability to live in the nuance of the gray area and acknowledge that life is full of uncertainty instead of allowing thinking traps to put you in places of extreme black and white thinking.

Oftentimes, when I say to people that life is full of uncertainty, the reaction I get, whether through their body language or facial expression, is of panic. The truth is, much of life has an element of uncertainty, and it's imperative that we learn to sit with this discomfort and self-soothe.

We need to learn to regulate our emotions when life feels incredibly unpredictable and uncertain.

As a parent, I notice that, whenever my daughter feels uncertain about an aspect of her life, she becomes anxious. This uncertainty can get her really worked up to the point where her head is spinning with these thinking traps. What I have noticed in my work with clients is that this anxiety and stress can happen regardless of our developmental stage. It does not matter whether you are in your twenties, thirties, forties, fifties or sixties, you can still fall into this trap of panic and anxiety when interfaced with the aspects of life that are full of uncertainty.

In these situations, realize that, while you can't control the outcomes, what you *can* control is the effort you put in. In order to make this shift and step into a high-powered mindset, you will need the flexibility to accept that life is, in fact, uncertain and develop a mindset that is balanced and not extreme.

SAY GOODBYE TO JUDGEMENT

With our fear of the uncertainty in life subsiding, it's important to recognize that a high-powered mindset does not use judgemental, absolute or harsh labels to describe the world, those in it, and of course, ourselves. What we want to do next is move away from these labels and develop a non-judgemental mindset.

This idea of using non-judgemental thinking and removing harsh labels not only applies to how you manage yourself and your perspective on an external level, but on an internal level, too. In other words, we need to monitor our self-talk. Pay attention to how you speak about others in your own mind. You might think that not sharing the negative things you think of others may be fine, but it's not. When you do this, you still fill your mind with judgemental thoughts, and this has the same level of toxicity as if you were to say it out loud. It takes a toll on your mental capacity and your ability to build resilience. I know you may feel like you are venting, even if it's just to yourself in your own mind, but it can still be harmful.

I want you to notice if this is happening and when it is happening. I want you to notice how it leaves you feeling, because I can almost guarantee that, at the core, it does not leave you feeling good. In fact, it may just leave you feeling drained and disempowered, and *this* is impacting your mindset.

Instead, what you want to begin practicing and implementing in your life is the use of language that is descriptive and includes the complexities and dynamic nature that exists in your world and relationships. You want to move your language away from the extremes and into a place of balance. I know I often talk about the gray area and the importance of staying in touch with the nuances of experiences and emotions, but it is important for your language to be nuanced, too, because a high-powered mindset is made up of beliefs and thoughts that make sense and are logical.

Questions for Self-Reflection:

φ What judgements am I applying to myself, to another person or to the world around me?

φ What is a more kind and compassionate way I can think instead?

My daughter is truly my biggest motivator to keep doing the work. I know that when I do my own inner work, I have the ability to give her the greatest gift I possibly can. I know that when I do my own work, I am able to show up for her, and I know you have at least one person, if not more, that you want to show up for.

When you dig deep to ensure that you carry high-powered beliefs, you are able to better show up for those that matter most, and it really is the most profound and beautiful expression of love and intimacy. When you strengthen the relationships with yourself and with others, you are able to see things about the relationship that perhaps were hazed before, and it really begins when you establish these guidelines for optimizing your high-powered beliefs. This is the key that will then lead you to a high-powered *lifestyle*.

THE HIGH-POWERED LIFESTYLE

Taking all these elements we have discussed and putting them into a framework you can commit to every day will allow you to maintain a lifestyle that is geared towards Emotional Mastery. Regardless of what areas you decide to change, if you do not commit to those practices and changes, you will revert back to old behaviors.

To ensure that your lifestyle is set up for success, you must also ensure consistency, congruency, and balance, which is approached with confidence. However, the reality is that, at times, you may be riddled with anxiety, and oftentimes, anxiety is the confidence killer.

For me, confidence and anxiety are highly correlated. In fact, anxiety can eat away at your confidence, which hinders your ability to master your emotions. The more anxious you feel, typically, the less confident you feel, and vice versa, the less anxious you feel, the more confident you feel.

LOOKING FEAR IN THE FACE

Let's look at the concept of fear, which is tied to anxiety. Whether it be because of a stressor in your life or because you are too focused on the things you can't control, what you will want to notice is that fear is at the core of anxiety. The problem with a fear-based life is that fear ultimately limits your choices. Fear makes you say no to certain opportunities or makes you isolate yourself, both of which can negatively impact your life.

Sometimes, fear and anxiety play into your relationships, too. Fear tells you what you should or shouldn't say, and teaches you to behave in very insidious ways. Fear and anxiety can dictate your choices and negotiate your relationships. Ultimately, fear is what traps you and leaves you feeling alone. Fear is the *real* culprit when it comes to your ability to live, love and communicate effectively.

Now, you may be asking yourself, "How do we combat this fear?" Well, the answer is by learning to manage it. By learning to manage your fear, you can reduce its impact on your mindset, which significantly increases your confidence and reduces your anxiety. It also increases your ability to communicate your needs and even connect with those you love.

Questions for Self-Reflection:

φ How much of what I am focusing on is aligning with fear?

φ What would happen if I traded in fear for faith?

This is why it is important to practice self-compassion and examine the thoughts and beliefs that plunge you into the dark areas you want to work on. When you look at the framework for success and becoming an Emotionally Intelligent Woman, the goal is to live a high-powered lifestyle where fear and anxiety are not killing your confidence, you understand that life has uncertainties and you value your own self-reflection and the feedback that you receive from others.

When you engage in these actions consistently, you will be able to see the transformations in yourself, your life and in your relationships that may have previously been defined by fear. When you reprogram your mindset at the level of your core beliefs, which lie within your subconscious mind, you unlock the ability to BECOME the woman who has the capacity to have the desires of her heart and achieve her goals. Even the ones that feel like they are bigger than you.

As I reflect on those years of being the only female expert on that TV show, I realize now that the process had nothing to do with achievement itself. It had nothing to do with the achievement of landing that gig, being asked back season after season or retiring with the rest of the crew. The process was all about me BECOMING the woman who could embody the desires of her heart, stand firmly in her mission and serve powerfully without fear. I may have appeared to have it all figured out on the outside, but on the inside, I was constantly doing my own inner work around reprogramming my core beliefs.

I had to do the mindset work, daily, in order to have the courage to show up. Instead of thinking the cameras were going to see right through me, I had to show up as the Emotionally Intelligent, confident woman I desire to be. I had to smile for the camera and really smile. I had to step into the shoes of a woman who believed she was worthy of her position in this world. And this is what I want for you. To become the woman who can hold the desires of her heart, achieve her goals and hold her position in the world.

Part Two

Communicate Fearlessly

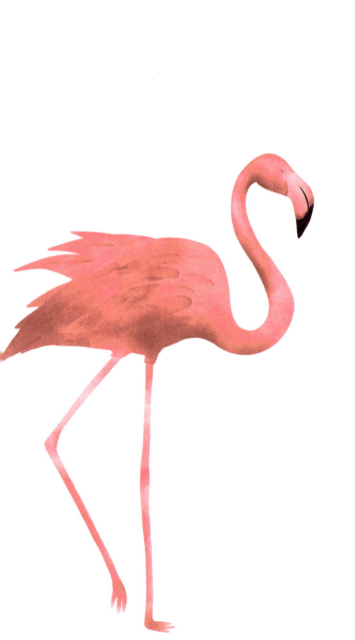

CHAPTER THREE

COMMUNICATION CULPRITS

"Cut out the culprits
and lay a foundation for
fearless communication."

I stood at the top of the stairs, taking deep breaths. I was finally going to tell him what I needed. I had rehearsed every single word I was going to say, and as I began walking down the stairs, within seconds of opening my mouth, he shut down. Immediately, I started crying, and ran back upstairs. This was one of those moments where I realized I couldn't do it anymore. I silently sobbed into a pillow in our bedroom, trying to hide my pain and frustration.

Conflict between my husband and I was (and still is) typically over relatively minor issues. Regardless of the mundane nature of our disagreements, I was often sent into an emotional spiral. It was never the *thing* we were arguing about that I would get fixated on, but *how we were communicating* with one another that would become the object of my fixation. The more I fixated on how we were "getting it wrong," the more emotionally dysregulated I would become.

I would become flooded with emotion. My face would be burning. My heart would be racing. I would get shaky and feel weak. In those moments, it was as if I couldn't hear or see anything. Then, next thing I knew, I would be in the bedroom upstairs, crying, again, while my husband would remain withdrawn in the living room. Then, he would come upstairs and go into the guest room for the night. That was *his* way of processing. Meanwhile, I couldn't sleep because my mind was still racing. I would be curled up in a ball under the covers, still dressed in my daytime clothes, pillow soaked in tears, waiting for him to engage with me. I would think to myself, "Healthy couples don't sleep apart. This is a bad sign. Next thing you know, we'll be headed for divorce." The thoughts would just come flooding in, and since neither one of us are prone to yell, it was deafeningly silent. It was always the silence that nearly broke me. I was flooded with all of these emotions, couldn't think straight, and couldn't communicate. Once I got into this vortex of emotion overload, I had no idea how to recover from it. I didn't even know how to go back to the conversation the next day and try again. I was truly lost.

It was this terrible spiral, with the next day feeling like a hangover. It was exhausting, and I was completely stuck. I would try to make sense of it and couldn't even remember how the conversation went or what we were actually in a disagreement about.

For many of the women I work with, the stories are similar. The content of the conflict between them and their partner may not be terribly significant, but they all feel a flood of emotion, nonetheless. In fact, it's the little things that become enormous in our heads. Despite my expertise in the areas of emotion regulation and communication, I couldn't seem to apply these skills in difficult conversations. I would get stuck in a really hostile place any time there was a disagreement and it would ignite in me this panic that having disagreements meant a bad relationship, and ultimately, the end of the world (a.k.a. catastrophizing). I had this fear-based tape replaying in my mind that disagreements, conflicts and disappointing one another was a huge sign that read: DANGER.

Then, began my surrender. And, my friend, it was a slow one as I was very stubborn to get there.

One of those nights when I was sleeping alone, I finally thought to myself, "I need to see a therapist." It was so hard for me to admit that I needed help with the very thing I helped others with for a living. The next day, I told my husband of my plans to get my own support. He didn't say a word, and you could cut the tension with a knife. At this point, money was really tight and I was on maternity leave, so it took every bit of courage to ask for support since I couldn't pay for it myself. It was difficult for me to admit that I needed help, and not only from a professional, but from him, too. I needed to communicate that to him, and even then, I didn't *ask* him. Instead, I said, "I am going to see a therapist. I made an appointment." The truth was, I had no clue how to ask for what I needed.

I did start seeing a therapist and continued working with her for many years. I recognized that, like many of the women I work with, I was struggling to communicate assertively and desperately needed to learn this critical life skill. My therapist and I worked through many things together: my thinking patterns, my communication style, my relationship style, and now, I see things very differently. One of the biggest shifts that came out of doing my own inner work was understanding that I was caught in, what I now call, Communication Culprits. I now knew that in order for me to communicate fearlessly, I would need to figure out how to get out of the new set of traps I had discovered.

TO COMMUNICATE FEARLESSLY YOU NEED TO IDENTIFY YOUR COMMUNICATION STYLE

When it comes to high-powered communication, the first step is to identify your particular communication style. There are four primary communication styles: the passive style, the aggressive style, the passive aggressive style, and the assertive style, and as we lay the foundation for fearless communication, we are going to dig deep into understanding the emotions that undergird these communication styles and look at the behaviors, the nonverbal cues and the subtle nuances that are associated with each. An important concept to keep in mind as we explore communication styles is that we learn how to communicate, primarily, from our family of origin.

THE PASSIVE STYLE: AVOIDING CONFLICT AT ALL COSTS

The passive style of communication is all about avoidance, which leads to resentment, and ends up with strained relationships. In other words, the passive style of communication is a vicious cycle of unmet needs, unresolved feelings and less than optimal relationship functioning.

If we have a passive communication style, quite simply, we try to avoid conflict at all costs. When passivity is our primary mode of moving through the world, we often feel anxious at the very thought of conflict, disagreement and even disapproval.

You have heard the term people pleaser, right? Well, this is the role that someone with a passive communication style would play. They please others at their own expense and doing so gives others control over them. Essentially, if your communication style is passive, you don't readily share how you feel, what you need or what you think. Instead, you may find yourself apologizing (for no good reason) and avoid expressing your opinions and disagreeing with others. You may even give into unreasonable demands from others and have a hard time sharing your thoughts or giving feedback. These are all indications of a passive communication style, and someone who struggles with a passive communication style does not want to do or say anything that may invite disapproval from others.

There are also less obvious clues that indicate someone has a passive communication style, and they are oftentimes nonverbal. If you have a passive communication style, you may make yourself appear as small as possible, speak softly, avoid eye contact, and carry a slouched body posture.

Some of these nonverbal cues were apparent in my mother growing up, and I vividly remember noticing them one day when my parents were on the phone having an argument. The conflict may have been about something small, but I remember it being enough to set my mother off for days. she had turtle into herself on the couch, speaking softly when spoken to and appearing small. It was something I witnessed multiple times growing up, and it was something that I found myself repeating as a new wife and mom. Part of my expertise is understanding one's family of origin and being able to discern the patterns that present themselves to allow for reprogramming of old scripts, but I was repeating patterns I had seen my mother have in my childhood. Seeing myself repeat old family of origin patterns was one of the hardest realizations I had had in my entire life and I didn't want to admit it to myself for a long time.

Every woman has likely said at one point or another, "I am not going to be like my mother," and I, personally, was putting so much pressure on myself to show up differently. When I realized I was communicating passively and exhibiting actions from my upbringing, I was very stubborn to accept it. It was very painful, and I vividly remember sitting in my therapist's office telling her how my absolute biggest fear wasn't being able to break those patterns. I remember having a conversation with my own mother about this fear of mine. We were on the phone and I asked her if she knew what my biggest fear was as a parent. She knew, and, understandably, it was hard for her to go there. To come face to face with what we know to be true: unless we make a concerted effort to change, we simply repeat patterns from our past. I told my mom how deeply afraid I was that my own inability to manage my emotions would keep me from having the sort of relationship I wanted with my daughter, and that if I didn't change by doing my own deeper work, I would repeat the patterns that would lead to relationship strain. That day, I also told my mom that I was determined to write a new narrative. One where I took radical responsibility for how I was showing up for the people that matter most.

My mother didn't have access to the support she needed when raising me and my younger siblings. I imagine she wanted things to be different, but access to training and support in Emotional Intelligence wasn't readily available at that time. I knew from making that realization that I would do anything I could to break free from those passive communication style patterns and learn a better way, not just for myself, but for my daughter.

When it comes to core beliefs, if you have a passive communication style, you may believe that the wants, needs and desires of others are more important than your own. Your mentality may be that others have rights and you do not, and others' contributions are valuable and yours are not.

I have experienced this firsthand. As a student, I really struggled with being passive. I wouldn't make contributions in class and I wouldn't engage in communication with my peers. I was just trying to quietly get through, and I did this up until I was getting my doctoral degree. In fact, it was *during* my doctoral degree that I made a concerted effort to break free from some of these patterns and began to contribute. The limiting belief I held was that my contributions were not as valuable as those of my peers and classmates. Eventually, I managed to shift my mindset so that I was able to feel confidence in myself and in my work. Once this happened, I began speaking up more easily and slowly began shifting my communication style.

What I have learned is that the struggle with passive communication style often originates from our family of origin. If you have a passive communication style, you may have grown up with a family that never really practiced saying 'no' or valued what 'no' meant. Perhaps, there were rules in your household that dictated you needed to be perfectly obedient, or there was a parental figure that set boundaries, but didn't respect anyone else's. In relationships like these, templates for assertive communication are not available because they were never modeled. If you didn't have the opportunity to see respectful, assertive communication between two people, then you have no framework to understand what that even looks like or understand that assertive communication is actually a very healthy way to communicate.

With a passive communication style, oftentimes, there is a deep fear of rejection and a feeling of helplessness that is undergirded by anger and frustration. You may even constantly feel you are being used by others, and with that, resentment begins to grow. Naturally, you will begin to experience a reduced sense of self-respect, which only further intensifies the tendency to use a passive communication style.

I want you to take note of when you might be falling into some of these traps and beliefs. I want you to realize that you are capable of much more and can break out of this toxic style of communication. It's difficult to feel confident and competent and have a sense of respect for yourself when you are unable or unwilling to communicate your needs, wants and desires clearly and congruently. In order to begin being more assertive, you will need to start by identifying your needs and wants and begin expressing them to others.

Questions for Self-Reflection:

φ How do I communicate with my family and coworkers?

φ How often do I apologize for things beyond my control?

THE AGGRESSIVE STYLE: A NEED TO MAINTAIN A SENSE OF CONTROL

The aggressive style of communication is marked by a need to maintain control and, often, to manipulate outcomes. While the aggressive style of communication does not always come across loud or physically threatening, it is undergirded by a need to maintain power, no matter what.

If you communicate with an aggressive communication style and navigate your relationships in this way, you have one goal in mind, and that is getting your needs met even if it's at the expense of others. You may feel you need to get what you want, have things go your way, and maintain a sense of control over others, regardless of what it costs you, the other person or the relationship.

Some of the characteristics of an aggressive communication style include the belief that your feelings and wants are superior to those of others and that any perspective other than your own is completely unreasonable or invalid. When stuck in the aggressive style of communication, you view the world in a very rigid, all or nothing sort of way. Essentially, if you have an aggressive communication style, your mindset is that you are always in the right and you tend to dismiss, ignore, or insult the needs, wants and opinions of others.

When it comes to more subtle, nonverbal cues, someone with an aggressive communication style may try to make themselves appear as big and threatening as possible. You may physically try to take up as much space as possible, regardless of how tall or big you actually are, make eye contact that is quite fixed and intense, and be unnecessarily loud.

It all really goes back to these ideas:

> φ *My contributions are more valuable than others*
>
> φ *My voice and opinion have greater value than others*
>
> φ *If others are afraid of me, they will make fewer demands of me*

Often, with this communication style, there is a power struggle, and while you may come across as extremely confident, the reality is that this behavior points towards very low self-esteem. The need to be aggressive in your relationships is driven by a fear that no one will really listen to you or take you seriously unless you communicate aggressively.

Similar to the passive communication style, the aggressive communication style is shaped within the family of origin. However, in this case, it is a different family dynamic. In many cases, someone with an aggressive communication style was likely raised by a parent who also displayed this communication style. In this household, it is possible that any small thing the child did would invite this aggression from the parent, which may have later taught that child to communicate in this way, and when people jumped and responded to what the child needed out of fear, the child felt a sense of satisfaction, only further encouraging this behavior.

If you have this style of communication, while you may feel your needs are being met, what you are really creating is a disconnection and lack of authenticity in your relationships. While you may feel you are getting your needs met in the short term, what is actually happening is an erosion of the very fabric of your relationships in the long term.

Often, an aggressive communication style shows up as anger, but underneath, what we are feeling is actually guilt. What happens at the end of the day is that we feel shame because we understand that we have hurt the ones we love, and while we have this realization, we get caught in the vicious cycle of communicating aggressively to keep getting what we want.

Questions for Self-Reflection:

φ Do I dismiss the thoughts and feelings of those around me?

φ How do I view myself compared to others?

THE PASSIVE AGGRESSIVE STYLE: A COMPLEX MIX OF EMOTIONS

A multi-layered communication style to work with is the passive aggressive communication style, and that is because it's a hard communication style to pinpoint and nail down. It's not as obvious as passive or aggressive communication styles, but is rather something that happens *in* relationships that may sometimes go unnoticed. It is a bit more complex, but the best way to put it is that it has similar characteristics to both the passive and the aggressive communication style. However, it is extremely subtle, covert and indirect.

If you have a passive aggressive communication style, you want everything to go your way without taking responsibility for your actions or your needs. Like the name suggests, it's a combination of passive and aggressive communication styles in which you want to get what you want at the cost of others, but don't directly ask or take responsibility for your requests. This communication style is covert, and is designed to soothe intense, unspoken anger while still getting your way, but without the openness and candidness of the aggressive communication style.

Given its complexity, if you have not already identified your communication style, you may be asking yourself if you communicate passive aggressively. Well, the behaviors of this communication style start with denial, something I have experienced myself. My husband would call me out on it, too. When I was snippy with him, he would immediately ask me what was wrong and say, "You might be stressed, but don't take it out on me." In the beginning, I would be immediately defensive. I would continue being snippy and say with an attitude and crossed arms that I wasn't taking it out on him. I was a hot mess, making demands without actually saying anything and being defensive and aggressive without even realizing it. If you find yourself relating to the passive aggressive communication style, don't be too hard on yourself. I didn't realize these behaviors until I really started to get honest with myself and actually listen and take into consideration what my husband was saying.

Another behavior that is common in the passive aggressive style of communication is avoidance. At the beginning of my relationship with my husband, there were times when I didn't want to socialize as much as he did. As an introvert and a bit of a homebody, I love my downtime, but instead of being honest and open with my husband, I had suddenly developed a "headache" and made up excuses as to why I couldn't go out. When I saw that this strategy had worked, whenever I didn't want to attend a social event, I would say I had a headache, stomachache or anything else to avoid going. While I don't do this anymore, it's important to note that the key here was the *intent*, and avoidance was a behavior I had become accustomed to getting what I wanted without explicitly asking for it. On some level, with the passive aggressive style of communication, we intend the negative outcome. We *intend* to feel bad, be late, forget, or whatever it is that allows us to avoid doing or whatever it is that we are in denial of. It's a matter of using denial, avoidance and excuses to get your needs met. Tricky, right?

These are the physical and verbal cues, but the less obvious, nonverbal cues can be just as indirect. These cues can look like those of someone with a passive communication style, but with stronger undertones of anger, resentment, or bitterness. Your needs may not be directly or overtly expressed, but people will get the hint of what it is you want through your actions, behavior and even tone of voice. Similar to the aggressive communication style, a core belief is a sense of entitlement. Even if you had made commitments or agreements to other people, deep down, you still have this belief that you are entitled to get your own way even if it means now denying the commitments and agreements that were made. Someone who has developed this style of communication probably has a history of using both passive and aggressive styles of communication. They might experience intense anger and a desire to control as well as a fear of expressing themselves directly. You also probably had parental figures that expressed combinations of passive and aggressive styles of communication that influenced your own.

What happens when you are passive aggressive is that there is often a fear of rejection if you are being too assertive and a strong sense of resentment at the demands of others. Over time, this evolves into even more resentment every time someone asks you to do something because you have no strategy for actually being assertive and become fearful of confrontation and your self-esteem plummets. Your anxiety also skyrockets because of the shame and guilt you feel of constantly letting others down. It's a continuous unhealthy cycle.

Questions for Self-Reflection:

φ Do I have difficulty asking for what I need directly from others?

φ Do I use indirect or manipulative strategies to get what I want??

THE ASSERTIVE STYLE: THE ONLY PATH TO FEARLESS COMMUNICATION, ELEVATED RELATIONSHIPS AND REAL CONFIDENCE

You may be asking yourself at this point which communication style will actually help deliver the kind of life and relationships you desire, and the answer is the assertive communication style. The assertive communication style is the ONLY style that increases personal power, confidence, and intimacy in relationships and helps high-powered women achieve their goals. The intent of this communication style is to maintain respect for others as well as respect for yourself and express yourself and your needs, feelings and ideas directly without feeling the need to be right at all times. Once practiced regularly, assertive communication is one of the most freeing ways to navigate your life and your relationships.

There is this sense of letting go of the outcomes and simply going with the flow while also respectfully addressing your boundaries. You hold ideas loosely and allow others to hold their own perspective without discounting or dismissing them, which is highly respectful. When it comes to nonverbal cues, something to be noticed with individuals who have an assertive communication style is they have very relaxed and casual body language and tend to be fluid in their movement as well as in their vocal quality. It is actually quite comfortable to be in a space with someone who communicates assertively because you feel respected and equal to this person. They provide frequent eye contact, but unlike the aggressive style of communication, this eye contact isn't intense or intimidating. Instead, it makes you feel seen and heard. Even their facial muscles and tone of voice seem relaxed and inviting.

With an assertive communication style, your core beliefs are not limiting, but rather, what I call, high-powered beliefs.

Here are some high-powered beliefs you can begin adopting so you can learn to communicate fearlessly and begin executing on the assertive communication style:

ϕ *Your needs and others' needs are of equal importance*

ϕ *You have just as much right to express yourself as anyone else*

ϕ *You are solely responsible for your own behavior*

I get really excited when I think about these high-powered beliefs because what I have learned is, when we are able to truly embrace these beliefs, we are able to take radical responsibility for our thoughts, feelings, and behaviors. It's amazing the impact a high-powered mindset has on us and our ability to truly change the landscape of how we communicate. If you begin navigating your relationships with an assertive communication style, you will see a radial improvement in your ability to master your emotions, respond to stressors and improve your overall sense of confidence. Communicating with an assertive communication style not only improves your personal self-image, but also your view of others and you will begin to feel really good about your interactions.

Now, this does not mean every single interaction you have once you develop an assertive communication style will be easy, or that you will get what you want. The purpose of assertiveness isn't about getting everything you want, it is about having the courage and the integrity to ask for it. The more you learn to navigate your relationships from a place of courage and integrity, the better you will feel about WHO you are and HOW you are showing up in your relationships. You will feel a sense of competence, like your contributions are valuable, and better understand where others are coming from. When you are assertive, you are better able to express your thoughts, needs and preferences without the expectation that others will automatically give in to you. You will be able to begin to understand how none of the other styles of communication are very satisfying to your life, let alone effective. In fact, none of them make space for openness, honesty or respect. From my own experience, assertiveness is truly the only way to really foster respect, openness and honesty in your relationships. It's the recognition that *you* are truly in charge of your own behavior and *you* are the driver of your choices.

Assertiveness may not come naturally to you, and you may want others to advocate for you, especially if you are afraid of conflict, but it is something you really need to practice. In fact, I would say assertive communication is a high-powered skill that leads to Emotional Mastery and living a limitless life. It is a skill that takes time, but the benefits it will bring to your life and relationships are worth challenging your already established and subconscious communication style. When you are able to communicate assertively, you will experience less conflict, anxiety and resentment. You will be able to focus on the present and be mindful and fully attuned in all of your relationships. You will be able to retain your self-respect, increase your self-confidence and reduce your need for the approval of others, and be fully and authentically engaged in your relationships.

Questions for Self-Reflection:

ɸ What beliefs get in the way of me communicating assertively?

ɸ What is a high-powered belief I can hold that will allow me to communicate fearlessly and embody the Emotionally Intelligent Woman?

An assertive communication style can dramatically improve your life, but it is crucial for you to do the mindset work and begin altering your core beliefs in order to build your assertiveness muscle. If you don't do the Emotional Mastery and mindset work first, you are not going to have the courage to have those difficult conversations. Now, for me, the biggest shift with my husband is I do the mindset work *before* I have the conversation with him. It's important to remember that the mindset work is not about getting what you want, but rather accepting that others' wants and needs are just as important and as valuable as your own. In the past, when I would ask my husband something, I would be so tied to the outcome that I would wind myself up so tight, but now I know better. Now, I know how to communicate honestly and get out of my own way, and because of this, there has been a huge shift in me. It was the first time in my life I was able to really communicate with my husband transparently about my needs and feel totally calm while doing it. I didn't know if he was going to give me what I was asking of him, but I knew I was completely responsible for my own happiness instead of putting that pressure on him. What an incredible feeling.

The crux of communicating fearlessly is reminding yourself that you can have the courage and integrity to ask for what you want, even if you cannot guarantee the outcome. It's about holding the reins of your own happiness because you know and understand that no one else can do it for you. It's about committing to having an assertive communication style and allowing yourself to begin developing an assertive mindset. When this happens, my friend, it is pure magic.

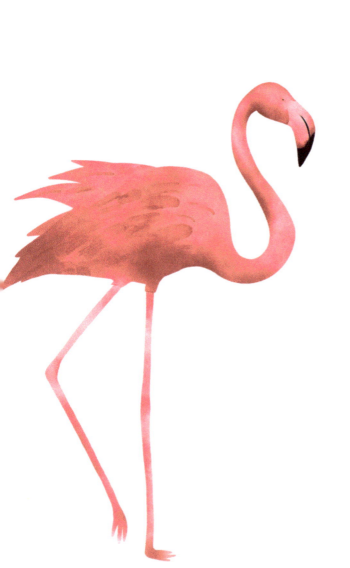

CHAPTER FOUR

THE ASSERTIVE MINDSET

"Become a boundary lover"

When I had dinner for the first time with my (now) husband's family when we were dating, I was amazed at their relationships. His parents were so direct with one another, and yet, somehow, no one seemed to be offended by the other. I never witnessed anyone getting defensive or feeling criticized. I remember someone boldly stated, "This tastes salty," and it was no big deal. Meanwhile, I was offended *for* the person who cooked the meal.

At the time, I remember wondering what it would be like to be able to communicate like that. Many years later, I have learned a lot about direct communication from my husband. When I met his family, I could see where he got his direct communication style from and why he does not become dysregulated by what others say. It was one of the first things that drew me to him. I found his ability to be open, honest and direct so attractive, and to be honest, rather liberating. His example of direct communication challenged me to step out of my comfort zone and radically change my mindset around communicating with others. I no longer wanted to hide out in my relationships. I wanted to speak assertively and establish boundaries. I became… a boundary lover.

There is a strong correlation between your ability to implement, set and maintain boundaries in your life and your ability to use an assertive communication style. One thing I have experienced and watched people get stuck in time and time again are boundaries. I have come to understand that a lack of boundaries often leads to a lack of *real* intimacy in relationships. In addition, a lack of boundaries creates an incredible amount of mental stress. In this chapter, we are going to unpack what boundaries are and their importance and connection to assertiveness, look at the number one thing that keeps people from actually setting boundaries, and look at how establishing and maintaining boundaries can actually lead you to an assertive mindset.

BALANCING TOGETHERNESS + SEPARATENESS = BOUNDARIES

When I talk about the concept of boundaries, I am not just talking about your personal relationships, but also your professional relationships and, really, any relationship you find yourself in. When you begin to define, negotiate and renegotiate boundaries in your relationships, you actually make space to engage with more authenticity. It's important to recognize that real intimacy isn't about being together and finding closeness all the time. Being together out of neediness or fear is, in fact, false intimacy.

Instead, real intimacy is the beautiful dance between togetherness and separateness. It's about finding the balance between the ability to be connected (together) and the ability to be apart (separate). This relational demarcation line can be drawn using boundaries. Even with romantic relationships, this balance and the use of boundaries are necessary. Without them, essentially, what ends up happening is you lose yourself in the relationship and the relationship suffers. In relationships that lack boundaries, people end up *not* showing up as their authentic selves, and instead, as shells of themselves. When you don't have boundaries in your life, you begin to feel anger, frustration and resentment. You lack a sense of personal agency, which makes it impossible to optimize your relationships and your mindset.

> *Real intimacy is not about being together and finding closeness all the time. Togetherness out of neediness or fear is, in fact, false intimacy. Instead, real intimacy is the beautiful dance between togetherness and separateness. It is about finding the balance between the ability to be connected and the ability to be apart. Boundaries are the gateway to this depth of intimacy.*

Even in parenting relationships, boundaries are critical. There was a time when I regularly delivered speaking events to parent communities at schools and one thing I would always let parents know was how important it was to set boundaries with their children. While some parents would look at me with disbelief, I knew setting boundaries with our children not only deepened our relationship with them, but actually helped them developmentally. Establishing boundaries with your children allows them to build confidence and resilience, which is what you ideally want for your children. A lot of parents, however, fail to set boundaries with their children out of fear, setting their children and the relationship up for distress in the future.

DON'T LET FEAR HOLD YOU BACK

Fear is ultimately what gets in the way of boundaries, and oftentimes, people are just deeply afraid of setting these boundaries. If you are struggling to set boundaries, if you are struggling to practice assertiveness, what is it you are afraid of?

What I have learned is that, often, we don't set boundaries because we are afraid of how others will react to them. We are afraid of being rejected or abandoned by the people we love. Mostly, we fear not being valued. Oftentimes, what keeps you in a passive style of communication is the idea that your self-worth and value are tied to your ability to do things for other people, but what I would like you to consider is that your self-worth and value are not at the hands of others, but up to you to determine. Assertiveness means you *set* boundaries in order to navigate your life, and I know it's not always easy, but this does not mean the boundary you are trying to set is a bad idea. It just means you might inconvenience the people around you that are pushing back on this boundary. They may not recognize or value the boundary you are trying to set, and this might invite some fear, but it's important to remain assertive and not go back on the boundary you are trying to set. Things will get worse before they can get better, and in order to have an assertive mindset and adopt a high-powered lifestyle, you need to set boundaries. You need to become a boundary lover.

Questions for Self-Reflection:

φ *If I begin to set boundaries, what am I afraid of?*

φ *If I begin to set boundaries, what do I stand to gain?*

ASSERT, PROTECT AND MAINTAIN YOUR BOUNDARIES

When you are setting boundaries, it's important to keep in mind that it's absolutely critical to assert, protect and maintain them. In reality, setting or asserting boundaries is really only half the battle. Protecting and maintaining those boundaries when people push back is the hardest component, and you must be prepared to do this. I really can't stress this enough, and here is why. If you set a boundary with someone and then fail to keep it, you will not be taken seriously, and you will begin to not take yourself seriously when it comes to setting boundaries. Take it from me, empty boundaries are bound to set you up for failure, so you need to protect and maintain them once you set them.

Questions for Self-Reflection:

> ϕ What boundaries do I need to establish with the people I love?
>
> ϕ What is something that really bothers me but I tend to shrug off?

TIMING IS EVERYTHING

When it comes to setting boundaries, timing is truly everything. You do not want to start getting assertive and setting boundaries when you are personally strained or going through an unusually stressful time. It just will not be an effective process. Instead, it is important to be intentional and reflective. Build up your resilience first.

Let's say you are planning on going away on a family vacation. In case it isn't obvious, this is not the time to be trying to set boundaries with the people you are going on this trip with. If you do, it may cause a strain on the relationship, the trip will not be very enjoyable and vacation is not a good reflection of everyday life. Instead, you want to select a time where you will have the courage, resources, *time*, and support to handle the pressures and pushbacks you are going to receive. If you don't select the timing correctly, you end up not being able to defend, protect and maintain the boundaries, placing you back at square one, letting others know that the boundaries you set can be broken and making it very difficult for you to renegotiate your relationships in the future.

Questions for Self-Reflection:

> ϕ When is a good time for me to establish this specific boundary with this person?
>
> ϕ Am I prepared to protect and maintain the boundary when/ if there is push back?

STAY STRONG

I know that reinforcing and maintaining boundaries is hard. It's harder than *setting* the boundary, but once you have selected your timing, you need to stay strong. You cannot back down, and this takes mental strength, support from others and self-care. If you don't remain strong when establishing these boundaries, especially for the first time, what is going to happen is that the people you are setting boundaries with are going to push harder next time. Then, you will find yourself in a vicious cycle of negotiating and renegotiating the same boundary with the same person over and over again, and that is not healthy for anyone involved. No matter how hard it gets, you must stay strong and stick to the boundaries you set. Like I said earlier, things will get harder and worse before they get easier and better, but in the end, you will thank yourself and you will come out of this with healthier relationship patterns and a high-powered mindset.

Questions for Self-Reflection:

φ Why is this boundary so important to me?

φ What is the cost of me not maintaining this boundary?

ONE RELATIONSHIP AT A TIME

The final piece I want you to remember when setting boundaries is to set them with one relationship at a time. This is so important; I can't stress it enough. You may be excited to implement all of these changes and actually renegotiate *all* the boundaries you have with your loved ones, but don't forget everything we have just talked about. Not everyone will be excited about you setting boundaries with them or will be accepting of the boundaries you are trying to set. Not everyone will react with kindness and be pleased if, suddenly, you become assertive and begin setting boundaries. The truth is, *you* probably will not be able to tolerate having all of your relationships strained and becoming difficult all at once. So, just pick one person and one relationship at a time.

The key here is to start with someone you think will be easiest to set boundaries with. Don't start with the most difficult person in your life in hopes of getting it out of the way quicker, and don't start with someone who is aggressive or passive aggressive. You don't want to start with the relationship you struggle with most because, if setting boundaries fails, and chances are it will, you may be less inclined to continue setting boundaries and you will revert back to your previous mindset and limiting beliefs. This is not the goal here. Instead, the goal is to become the best version of ourselves, the Emotionally Intelligent Women we know we can be, living high-powered lifestyles. Therefore, start with the easiest person to set boundaries with. Now, this relationship does not need to be a personal one, it could be a professional relationship with a coworker or colleague, but it just needs to be someone whom you think is not going to give you a hard time for establishing these boundaries.

Questions for Self-Reflection:

ϕ Who is the hardest person for you to imagine setting boundaries with?

ϕ Who is the easiest person for you to imagine setting boundaries with?

In all honesty, I don't think setting boundaries ever becomes easy, but we become more comfortable with the discomfort of boundary setting the more boundaries we set and slowly begin building our confidence.

Now, you may be asking yourself, "HOW exactly do I begin setting these boundaries?" The answer is, as you move through different developmental stages in your life, you move through different levels of over-functioning, which simply means doing more than what is reasonably required in a given relationship. If you are struggling to set boundaries, feeling overwhelmed, or heading towards burnout, you are probably over-functioning in several of your relationships. This is why it is so important to continuously audit your relationships and your fears to determine if they are getting in the way of setting boundaries. I want you to take a close and critical look at all of your relationships and your tendency to over-function. Have an honest look at your fears and begin implementing some of the high-powered beliefs needed to elevate your relationships. Look at your core beliefs and communication style. What is benefiting you and what is hindering you?

ACTUALLY COMMUNICATE

The single biggest problem in communication is the illusion that it has taken place when it has not. How often have we walked away from conversations thinking one thing of it when the other person thought something else? We often forget that communication is not only a two-way street, but also occurs on a variety of different levels with both verbal and nonverbal cues involved.

Ask yourself this:

φ *What relationships and conversations do I need to return to?*

φ *What have I missed in these conversations and relationships?*

φ *Where are those areas in my life that require me to modify and hone my communication skills?*

With these questions answered, on paper or in your head, I want you to remind yourself that you are in charge of your own behavior and the driver of your choices. You do not need to justify yourself to others or ask for their approval, just like others do not have to justify themselves to you or ask for your approval. In that same vein, you are not responsible for others' problems, just like others' are not responsible for yours. When you are direct and assertive, you open the door to better communication, understanding, and overall, relationships with the people in your life. It will not be an easy shift, and it's important to allow yourself room for error, but remember your timing, effort and dedication. Start slow and you will see all the benefits that come with establishing boundaries and adopting an assertive mindset.

Eight months after that dinner with my husband's family where I was horrified *and* intrigued by their assertiveness, he proposed. I had not been expecting it all and, and I am so grateful to now be married to a man who challenges me to be direct and assertive. I am grateful that I got to witness how direct and assertive his family is with each other because it moved me to step out of my passiveness and step into the shoes of a woman who understands the needs and wants of others without belittling her own. In order to adopt an assertive mindset, you need to put in the mindset work and realize that conflict is okay. In fact, it is healthy. People are not always in agreement with one another, and that is okay. You need to establish boundaries and work on your communication skills so you can deepen your relationships with authenticity and honesty. Trust me, it's incredibly rewarding to see how the changes you make for yourself can have such a positive impact on your life and can lead you to become a better version of yourself.

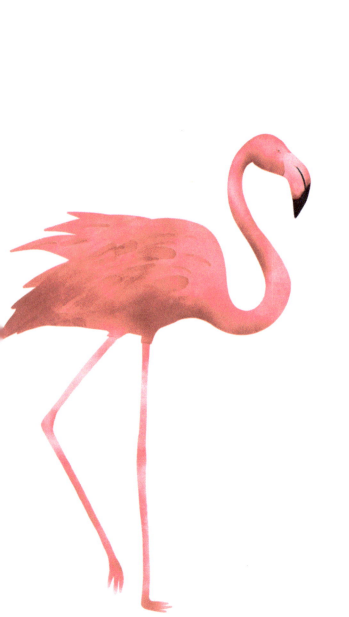

CHAPTER FIVE

THERE ARE EMOTIONAL NEEDS, THEN THERE ARE EMOTIONS AND NEEDS

"You are the boss of your emotions. They work for you."

I t took me a while to realize *I* was the one getting in the way of my own relationship with my husband. Before I did my own Emotional Mastery work, before I looked inward and saw that a lot of the stress I had put on the relationship was coming from my unspoken expectations and limiting beliefs, I really thought my inability to show up was because of something outside of myself. I felt all of these different emotions that were causing me to spiral in my relationships without ever realizing what my needs were. It wasn't until I began peeling through the deeper layers that I got to the core of what I needed and how I could better show up and actually communicate my needs with clarity. With that said, I want you to ask yourself this. Have you ever thought that maybe *you* were the one who was getting in your own way? Have you ever thought that maybe it's *your* unspoken expectations and limiting beliefs that are holding you back from becoming the Emotionally Intelligent Woman you want to be?

Truthfully, it's an ongoing journey, and I still continue to do the work daily. Reading this book is not going to automatically turn you into an Emotionally Intelligent Woman, but it will provide the stepping stones you need to become committed to mastering your emotions and have the courage to really transform your life. It's a constant process of leaning in and having difficult conversations and challenging beliefs you have always had, but once you begin showing up for yourself, it becomes easier to show up for others. Instead of thinking that emotions are what *run* you, consider that *you* are the boss of your emotions. They do not define you. They work for you. There is a lot of work that goes into becoming an Emotionally Intelligent Woman, and one of the components we need to look at is emotion itself. Emotions and needs go hand in hand and are incredibly critical components to communicating fearlessly and elevating your relationships. As you move through this chapter, you are going to have a really good understanding of emotions and how to regulate them. You are going to be able to differentiate between your emotions and your needs and actually begin having difficult conversations with yourself and the ones you love.

EMOTIONS AND NEEDS GO HAND IN HAND: THE ROLE OF EMOTIONS

Your emotions provide you with incredibly valuable information about your needs and can help to inform your assertive communication. They are informative guides that help you to navigate your interactions with others and inform you of when you need to assert yourself. When you think about your emotions, and are able to identify what you are feeling, you dramatically increase your ability to be self-aware. This self-awareness is necessary to becoming the Emotionally Intelligent Woman you want to be. Emotions also play a key role in developing empathy, which is what allows you to connect with others and is truly the crux of any healthy relationship. Empathy, in essence, is feeling felt by another person. It's that whole idea of *I feel you*, and your personal level of awareness is directly correlated with your ability to be empathetic in relationships. Essentially, in order to empathetically understand others, you must start by developing a deep awareness of your own emotions and the impact they have on you.

Emotions also tell us what our likes and dislikes are and help us navigate comfort and discomfort. They give you information about your response to situations and establish your preferences. I want you to begin using the language of preferences as you navigate the different places and relationships that make up your life and become aware of the times in which you are reactive to your emotions rather than responsive. When you are not self-regulated and have not mastered your emotions, you can begin to feel anxious in your relationships, which is why it is crucial to understand the emotions you are feeling before reactively engaging in your relationships with others. Along with your thoughts, your emotions give you information on what you like, want and need. Truthfully, I don't think you can begin practicing assertiveness without actually identifying your emotions, and here is why: in order to be able to practice assertiveness, you need to be able to self-regulate, and the very first step of self-regulation is emotional awareness.

Questions for Self-Reflection:

φ What emotions am I experiencing?

φ What facts am I deciding not to look at because I am favoring how I am feeling?

IT'S JUST (PRIMARY AND SECONDARY) EMOTIONS TAKING ME OVER

Now, like many other things, emotions are not simply black and white. There are primary and secondary emotions, and these two types of emotions impact one another. A primary emotion is the very first emotion that is *actually* triggered within us. Typically, primary emotional triggers leave us feeling vulnerable, helpless or powerless. They are the emotions that emerge in uncomfortable situations, difficult conversations or in relationships that are strained. Then, secondary emotions are the emotions that are openly expressed and that we would be most familiar with or most aware of. The role of the secondary emotion is to *protect* the vulnerability that is being triggered by the primary emotion. Think of it this way. Picture an iceberg. Secondary emotions are the emotions we can see. They are the tip of the iceberg, the emotions that are visible on a surface level. Then, primary emotions lie beneath the water. they are the emotions you have suppressed deep down. These might be the emotions you have been told growing up not to express or the ones that leave you feeling so vulnerable that you have trained yourself to ignore. Primary emotions are the emotions you carry very deep inside, but ultimately, it is your secondary emotions that come through and act as reactions to your primary emotions.

A movie I have watched countless times with my daughter is *How the Grinch Stole Christmas*. If you have not seen it, go watch it. It's a great movie, and the reason why I'm sharing it with you is because it relates to primary and secondary emotions. If you know the storyline, it's all about the Grinch, and he's angry, resentful, and overall, quite hateful towards others. The Grinch doesn't want to be around people and isolates himself up in his mountaintop cave with his dog Max. Now, the people of Whoville are ultimately terrified of the Grinch and they all experience the Grinch as angry, but while they think anger is the Grinch's primary (and only) emotion, really, the anger they see is his secondary emotion. As you go through the storyline, you see, close to the end, that it all reels back to his childhood. You begin to see that, when the Grinch was young, he was bullied and picked on for looking different. He was green, with fur everywhere, unfitting the norm. Looking back to his childhood, you begin to realize and understand that the Grinch isn't angry at the world, but rather he's sad and hurt at how his peers treated him. This makes the Grinch's primary emotion sadness even though the tip of the iceberg points to anger. This example is something I talk about often with my daughter. We'll often use the phrase "Do you remember how the Grinch's sadness turned to anger?" It's the way I have taught her to understand the difference between primary sadness and secondary anger, in this case. The Grinch was actually really loving and loyal, but in that place of vulnerability, he was really hurt and had to carry a great deal of sadness for a long time, which he presented as anger because he couldn't tolerate feeling sad any longer.

What happens in real life is just like the story of the Grinch. We all have primary emotions that are very vulnerable, sometimes even raw, and can leave us feeling powerless. If we experience and stay with these emotions for long enough, we fear that they will break us. We can only tolerate the discomfort of those primary emotions for so long without a way of processing them. This is why we develop secondary emotions to protect us from the vulnerability being triggered by the primary emotions we are feeling. Some emotions are more readily accessible and identifiable than others, and we are more likely to identify and express emotions we are comfortable with. Just like the Grinch dealt with shame, fear and pain and suppressed these uncomfortable emotions, we are more likely to suppress uncomfortable emotions too. As women, interestingly enough, the emotion we tend to suppress is actually anger, which is, for many of us, a primary emotion. Anger invites us to feel powerless and vulnerable, which brings up a secondary emotion that is meant to be protective.

I want you to really think about this: what are the emotions that others see you express? These emotions are quite likely not your primary emotions, which are at the core of your experience and the emotion actually in charge. Primary emotions often present themselves as criticism, blame and irritability, which we don't necessarily want others to see, and while they are under the surface, primary emotions are the ones that drive our choices, actions and behaviors, and if we don't get a handle on this, we'll continue to be reactive and fail at mastering our mindset.

Questions for Self-Reflection:

φ What emotion(s) do I typically project outward?

φ What are the most vulnerable emotions I experience that I may be suppressing?

THOUGHTS AND EMOTIONS ARE NOT THE SAME THING

In order to appropriately identify our emotions, we need to be able to discern the difference between our thoughts and our emotions. Now, it is really important to clearly understand that emotions and thoughts are not the same. While they are absolutely connected and influence one another, there is a very distinct difference between them, and I have a formula that could help:

WHEN X HAPPENS, I FEEL Y BECAUSE I THINK Z.

I want you to think of an emotion, and then, I want you to think of a situation or event that triggers that emotion. For example: when **my partner does not answer my text right away (situation)**, I feel **anxious (feeling)**, because I think **he does not care (thought)**.

While we tell ourselves that it's the situation that drives our feelings, this isn't an accurate understanding of how our emotions operate. It's in fact our thoughts that drive our feelings about any given situation. The situation does not trigger the feeling, the thought you have about the situation is what triggers the feeling.

Use the formula above to get crystal clear and concrete about what it is you are saying to yourself that is triggering your feelings so that you can better master your emotions.

Another distinction to consider is that simply putting the words "I feel" in front of a statement does not make it a feeling. I will give you a more specific example. Let's look at the statement "You don't care about me." Have you ever said this to someone you love at one point or another? In this instance, putting "I feel" in front of "You don't care about me" does not make it a feeling. In this instance, "You don't care about me" is a thought, not a feeling. Just because you put "I feel" in front of a statement does not necessarily make it a feeling. It's more complex than that. In the example of "You don't care about me," the best way to express this statement is to say "When you don't answer my text, I feel anxious, because I think you don't care about me," because this is a thought *you* have that drives the feeling of anxiety.

With emotions and thoughts, there comes this mess of rambled ideas, but it does not have to be this way. When my husband and I were beginning to get more serious in our relationship, I would feel upset when he didn't call me during the workday. I would *think* he didn't care about me and mistake this thought for an emotion. Once I began working on mastering my emotions, instead of associating him not calling with the thought of him not caring, I realized that was simply a thought in my head and worked to change it rather than let it dictate my emotions, and, ultimately, my self-image. I was showing up and making the decision that I wasn't going to let my thoughts get the best of me and trigger maladaptive emotions.

Questions for Self-Reflection:

φ • What are the maladaptive emotions I experience most regularly?

φ • What are the thoughts I am saying to myself that are driving those emotions?

I AM THE DECISION-MAKER OF MY EMOTIONS, NOT THE OTHER WAY AROUND

Decision-making is a key concept when it comes to Emotional Intelligence, and emotions can either help our decision-making or get in the way. We now have clarity that emotions play an important role in our lives, but have you ever considered the influence that your emotions have on your decision-making? Believe it or not, decision-making is a behavior, and our thoughts drive our emotions, which drive our behavior, and it's really important to understand the tremendous impact here. Whatever we think, whatever we are saying in our heads, this perspective is what is going to drive our emotions. So, if our thoughts are negative, it's going to drive negative emotions, which are then going to drive negative behaviors, choices and actions.

What we want is to establish a healthy, high-powered mindset, because if our mindset is optimized and our thoughts are filled with high-powered beliefs, then it's going to drive healthy emotions, like confidence, happiness, and joy, which will dictate the way we make decisions. Even if our mindset is filled with positive, high-powered beliefs, it's still important to not make decisions solely based on emotions. When we do this, it's almost like we have got blinders on, and we run the risk of losing sight of the full picture and diminishing and narrowing our perspective. When we react and act solely based on our emotions, we create a reality for ourselves that may not reflect true reality. For example, if you are feeling jealous and suspicious and automatically assume your partner is cheating on you, you may make some irrational decisions about the relationship or allow this thought to drive up your anxiety. Even if it contradicts your current feelings, it is important to look at things clearly and see all the information you have before making irrational decisions based on thoughts and emotions.

Clearly, I believe that emotions are important. They are instructive and give us incredibly valuable information, but what can happen, from a cognitive perspective, is that we can focus on emotions in the absence of reasoning. This becomes incredibly problematic when making decisions because the more you solely rely on your emotions to make decisions, the more your anxiety goes up and your ability to make decisions goes down. It's critical to become aware of this and begin making decisions from a rational place, which will make you feel more confident. I want you to remember that while emotions are instructive, they shouldn't be driving your decision-making. It's imperative that you truly understand your emotions so that you can fully execute and own your decisions. You need to be the boss of your emotions, not the other way around. You need to take radical responsibility for all the parts of your life, including your emotions and your ability to make decisions.

Questions for Self-Reflection:

φ *How do I react when I am giving into a negative thought?*

IT'S TIME TO GET EMOTION-SMART

To increase our Emotional Intelligence, we need to expand our emotional language and, in turn, our emotional awareness. It's really all about getting clear about the emotions both beneath the surface and at the tip of the iceberg. People who run from us when we get sad, angry or afraid also run from themselves when they get sad, angry, or afraid, so don't take it too personally. It is so often that we take people's choices personally when it has little or nothing to do with us in the first place. Always keep in mind the humanness, the journey and the limitations of the people you are in relationships with. We each come to the process of change at our own time, and right now, I want you to focus on where you are and where you are headed. When we struggle with our emotional regulation, or even emotional awareness, we limit our capacities to respond well in conversations, and I want you to have a really good look at what is at the tip of your emotional iceberg and what lies beneath that level of awareness. Trust me, it will take you a long way and help you to self-regulate and get into the position of living a high-powered lifestyle as an Emotionally Intelligent Woman.

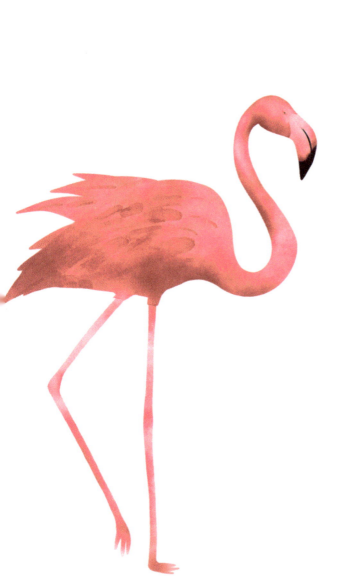

CHAPTER SIX

R.E.A.L TALK

*"It's not what you say,
it's how you say it.*

"**M**ommy, why does your vagina look different from mine?"
I was putting my daughter to bed when she asked me this
question during our snuggle. At first, I was taken back.
She asked without shame or any hesitation, something that was very new
for me based on my old narratives around women's bodies and sexuality.
I explained to her that, as females, all parts of our bodies are unique and
different, including our vulvas and vaginas. Still stuck on the subject, I
grabbed my phone and shared with her an educational image that my good
friend who is a sexual health expert posted on her Instagram feed on the
very topic. My daughter was surprised to learn that social media could be
used to educate women about their bodies. While the conversation was
unexpected, it was amazing, and to think that it started with vaginas and
ended with the importance of educating women in all areas of life. It was

amazing that I was able to engage with her so openly, feeling equipped to have the conversation. I remember the interaction about sexuality being vastly different from the ones I experienced growing up, and it was in that moment that I realized I was redefining a relationship template. I was so proud. It wasn't about *what* I was saying, but about *how* I was saying it, and that makes all the difference.

My daughter is my why. Motherhood is my greatest mission. As much as I love my work, it pales in comparison to my calling to lead with love, integrity and intentionality in my daughter's life. To show up well for her is my deepest desire and greatest goal, and before this realization, becoming a mom was truly my biggest fork in the road. Motherhood was my wake-up call and my greatest turning point, and I am grateful for it. I truly believe, with every fiber of my being, that if I had not had my daughter, if it had not been for her, I would still be stuck in my old ways. I would still be feeling sorry for myself, playing the victim, not taking responsibility for my own actions and happiness, and blaming other people for my problems. If it wasn't for my daughter, I would still be emotionally immature. I would have been nowhere close to showing up as the best version of myself for the person who needed me the most. So, I want you to take a moment and reflect on the answers to these questions. Who needs you the most? Who needs you to show up as your best self? Who needs you to do your own work so that you can lead with love, integrity and intentionality? When you know the answers deep in your heart, it will be the force that drives you to the transformation of becoming the woman you are called to be in this world.

It's time to get **R.E.A.L.**, which is how I want to help you become the Emotionally Intelligent Woman I know you can be. R.E.A.L. is a formula I created to help you communicate with confidence and begin building a high-powered lifestyle. It's a formula based on four elements that go hand in hand in helping you to practice and master your emotions, so you can communicate with the utmost confidence.

Regulating emotions

Expressing needs

Accepting outcomes

Letting go

You can think of this formula as a tool for planning and executing difficult conversations, asking for what you want and setting boundaries.

LET'S GET R.E.A.L: REGULATE EMOTIONS

Learning to regulate your emotions is a critical skill when it comes to Emotional Mastery *and* communicating fearlessly. It's about being mindful and learning to identify your emotions without feeling ashamed of them and without putting them onto others.

FEEL YOUR EMOTIONS, NAME YOUR EMOTIONS

When it comes to regulating emotions, Dan Siegel, an interpersonal neurobiologist, teaches us that there is incredible power in the simple practice of naming our emotions. When we begin to name our emotions, we begin to expand our emotional awareness and emotional language. So, the first step to naming our emotions is simply becoming aware of them. Once aware, we can begin identifying them and naming them. It's a matter of learning to master our emotions rather than having them master us.

This is something that I needed to be constantly aware of when learning to master my own emotions. I needed to remember that I couldn't allow my emotions to control me, no matter how intense or overwhelming they were, and this is critical to the assertiveness framework. When assertiveness is not a practiced skill, it often brings with it a lot of difficult emotions, and that is why a great place to begin the practice of emotional regulation is simply with naming our feelings.

Imagine feeling both fear and courage as you step into your mission of becoming your best self. These are two very powerful constructs, and I have felt both of them many times in my life. We know that the majority of leaders struggle with imposter syndrome and self-doubt, and oftentimes, this is at the hand of fear. Each time I make a change, take a risk, and decide to play a bigger game, I am flooded with the fears that undermine my sense of confidence, but fear is never a good indicator that you are headed in the wrong direction. In fact, fear is a normative part of what it is like to move closer to your personal mission, and I have witnessed this firsthand. I had spent most of my adult life gathering credentials to hold the title of psychotherapist, graduating from my doctoral degree when I was two and a half months pregnant with my daughter. I had spent the last two decades, dedicated to my craft, in service to my own calling and to the lives of those I was helping. Then, February 22nd, 2021, was the day I had my very last session as a psychotherapist, and began pouring my energy into a new direction. I would have never imagined that, when I started my journey as a psychotherapist, I would meet a fork in the road in my 40s, "retiring" from a title I had worked so hard to achieve . It was scary for me to walk away from the professional title that had given me such a powerful sense of identity and to begin the work of redefining myself without the immediate respect that comes with it. It was terrifying for me to listen, intently, to the call within my heart that was telling me my life was meant for so much more. As scary as it was to say goodbye to a very powerful part of my identity, I left my one-on-one practice, not because I was ready, but because my mind could no longer ignore what I was feeling deep inside my heart. I needed to identify that emotion, name it 'fear' and see that it was simply a feeling that came with the change that was needed.

On a very deep level, I knew I wanted to continue working with people, but in particular, I wanted to work with women in a more immersive and transformative way. I wanted to be able to ask questions like, "Have you ever felt like your life is meant for more? Are you making space for your growth and your personal expansion or are you believing lies about your worth and capacity of contribution? What if you stopped playing small and allowed your mind to expand enough to contain the hopes and dreams your heart has already captured? What if you gave yourself the permission to go all in on who you are, who you are called to be and what your mission is in this world?" In order to show up as the woman I knew I was meant to be, I had to identify all the different emotions I was feeling and regulate them. I had to name my fear 'fear' for me to overcome it and continue on my journey of becoming an Emotionally Intelligent Woman.

Questions for Self-Reflection:

φ **What emotions am I feeling? What are their names?**

CONQUER FEAR WITH MINDFULNESS

Mindfulness is a concept we hear so much about these days, and it's a concept with a significant impact on our ability to manage our moods. One of the experts on mindfulness, Jon Kabat-Zinn, an American professor emeritus of medicine and the creator of the Stress Reduction Clinic and the Center for Mindfulness in Medicine, Health Care, and Society at the University of Massachusetts Medical School, defines mindfulness as "the awareness that arises through paying attention, on purpose, in the present moment, non-judgmentally." There are a few components that make up mindfulness, but it really starts with slowing down to connect with your body. It's being intentional and purposeful, and remaining in the present moment while taking on an attitude of non judgement. Essentially, it's the regular practice of really just being with yourself and your emotions, and you will be amazed at what a difference it makes in increasing your emotional awareness.

When you practice mindfulness, you allow thoughts and feelings to flow through you without needing to change or judge them. If you have never practiced mindfulness, this may actually be a little harder than you think, and it's astounding how self-critical you can be when it comes to your own thoughts and feelings. It is something that certainly requires practice, but when mindfulness invites you to remain in the present, it also invites you to remain in your body, connected to your breath and in the moment rather than in the past or in the future. When you find yourself caught in thinking traps, what these thinking traps are really doing is pushing you into the past or into the future. Mindfulness is the best antidote as it increases your self-awareness. In order to manage fear, or any other negative emotion that you have named and identified, you need to practice mindfulness and allow yourself to feel the emotion without holding onto it.

Questions for Self-Reflection:

φ *What would it be like to slow down and practice a more mindful approach to your emotions?*

φ *Are there emotions you might be hesitant to acknowledge?*

BE RESILIENT TO YOUR SHAME

One emotion that will absolutely try to hijack our ability to self-regulate and sabotage our relationships is shame. Just like we need to be aware of all our emotions, we need to increase self-awareness around shame. Now, shame and guilt are often put together, but it is important to differentiate these two emotions. Shame is the deeply painful experience of not feeling good enough or worthy of love. It's a very deep sense of inadequacy and completely immobilizes us, making it impossible for us to communicate our needs in our relationships. In truth, shame is the single most toxic emotion that can absolutely wreak havoc on our lives, destroying any inclination to practice assertiveness. This is why shame resilience is so critical, because when we are plagued with shame, we develop this idea that we are undeserving of having our needs met. There is really no way to begin setting boundaries and communicating with confidence when we feel shame because of the deep, powerful, negative narrative it creates in our minds.

I want you to take a moment and ask yourself if you are struggling with this. Does this resonate with you? Do you find yourself telling yourself you are undeserving of having your needs met? If you find yourself constantly stuck in a cycle of not being able to practice being assertive and setting boundaries, you most likely have some work to do in building your shame resilience, and that is okay. You are not alone. Shame is a universal experience triggered by a variety of common life experiences. Failure, to some degree, is a trigger to shame, but it's important to remember that we all make mistakes. Maybe, at some point in your life, you experienced emotional or verbal abuse, or even in some cases, physical abuse. I have yet to meet a human being that has not experienced the pain of rejection, and it's these experiences that contribute to the universal experience of shame.

Here is the thing I want you to really understand about shame. Shame is ultimately caused by a threat to your idealized identity. It's essentially what happens when something challenges the way you prefer to view yourself or how others perceive you, and this idea of an ideal identity holds true for everyone. Most women hold an idealized identity around being a good mother, partner or daughter, and I, for one, have certainly struggled with holding an idealized identity around all three. I always wanted to be a good daughter for my parents and make them proud. Then, when I got married, as a registered couple and family therapist, I, of course, wanted to be a good partner. After that, the idealized identity followed me into motherhood, and I told myself that I wanted to be a good mother, too. I really wanted to nail this idealized identity but of course, I wasn't able to and began feeling shame. Anything that threatened this idealized identity I was trying to create for myself, like hearing my daughter tell me when she was upset that I was an awful parent or even failing her at something, made me very vulnerable to shame.

We all have idealized identities that we would like to live up to, but it's important to remember we can't live up to those expectations 100% of the time. This need for perfection is a thinking trap that contributes to your feelings of shame and gets in the way of your shame resilience, which is so important to your mindset mastery. It's important to remember that we are all, as human beings, flawed and imperfect. It's important to put your best foot forward and become resilient to the shame that tries to take you over.

Questions for Self-Reflection:

φ *In what areas of my life do I experience shame?*

φ *How does shame hold me back?*

DON'T LET YOURSELF SUFFER

Now, the reason I keep bringing up Emotional Mastery is because it is designed to equip you with the tools necessary to regulate your emotion, and sometimes, to regulate your emotions, you need to challenge your thinking. This is where cognitive reframing comes in.

Cognitive reframing is basically taking your thinking and challenging it in order to develop high-powered beliefs. Now, there is a quote by Haruki Murakami, a Japanese writer, that I really love that can help you to understand a little more about cognitive reframing, and it goes, "Pain is inevitable, but suffering is optional." For me, this is entirely true. Pain is inevitable, and we are all going to experience it at some point, but suffering, on the other hand, is completely optional. Suffering is a state of mind you put yourself in. So, in order to master your emotions, essentially, what you need to do is challenge your thinking by reminding yourself that suffering is indeed optional and pain is indeed inevitable. It's in your hands. How you respond to pain is on you, and through cognitive reframing, we are able to move towards assertive communication, entirely shifting our perspective, all by just training our brains.

LET'S GET R.<u>E</u>.A.L: EXPRESSING YOUR NEEDS

To effectively communicate, you need to realize that we are all different in the way we perceive the world and use this understanding as a guide for how you communicate with others. Each and every one of us has a unique perspective, understanding and experience of the world around us, and it's important to remember that your perspective is simply *your* perspective. Just because you see things in a particular way does not mean that others will see it in this way, too. So, the more space you make for multiple perspectives, the easier it becomes for you to navigate your relationships with confidence and love and express your needs and understand the needs of others.

LEARN TO COMMUNICATE

In order to truly express your needs, you need to be able to communicate them clearly and assertively, but sometimes you may not really know what it is you need. If you have never had the opportunity to slow down and identify what your needs are, it becomes extremely difficult to express them. Furthermore, if you have gone a long time operating out of a passive, aggressive or passive aggressive communication style, you really don't even know how to express your needs clearly and congruently, and this is where you can become really stuck.

Communication is, essentially, assertiveness in action. It's really important to remember that communication is not just words, but a combination of words, body language, tone of voice and non-verbal cues. Sometimes, we can communicate without saying anything, and in fact, roughly 90% of communication does not come from words, but rather from so-called silence. Communication is really a combination of what is said and not said and what is done and not done. I mean, do you know if your partner is angry just by the way they walk through the door when they get home? Maybe, it was the way they opened the door or slammed the cabinet door. All of these nonverbal cues contribute to communication, and a combination of secure attachment style and high-levels of differentiation allow you to communicate assertively.

Questions for Self-Reflection:

ϕ How can I better communicate what I am feeling and what I need?

ϕ What would it be like to communicate assertively?

STRENGTHEN YOURSELF AND COMMUNICATE YOUR NEEDS WITH CONFIDENCE

You already know confidence plays a role in your ability to communicate in general, but confidence is also critical to your ability to express your needs. Assertive communication is really contingent on your ability to build confidence, and unfortunately, there are thinking traps that truly are confidence killers and anxiety provokers. For you to be able to express your needs confidently and practice assertiveness, it's crucial that you manage and monitor your confidence killers and anxiety provokers because when these thinking traps eat at our confidence, it erodes, and so does your assertive communication.

The purpose of optimizing assertiveness is to express your needs with confidence, but when your foundation is feeling weak and requires reinforcements, it's important to exercise your high-powered mindset and be mindful of what you need to do to show up for yourself and be better. Take the time to strengthen yourself and strengthen your foundation. Now, it's perfectly normal to need reinforcements on all these concepts. If you feel that confidence killers or anxiety provokers are coming back for you, check your foundation and exercise your confidence muscles, even if you don't feel like they are there to begin with. Trust me, they are.

COMMUNICATION MUST BE H.O.T.

Dan Oswald, the author of *The Oswald Letter, Insights on Business and Leadership* and CEO of Business & Legal Resources, Inc., says communication should always be H.O.T. that is honest, open and two-way, and this is a great little acronym to keep in mind. It's also important to keep in mind that you must not be *emotionally* hot when having difficult conversations. The point here is that, if you want to build amazing relationships and communicate fearlessly, it's going to require that you go to some tough places in those relationships. Authentic human connections are the key to personal and career success, and they aid in your showing up as an Emotionally Intelligent Woman. You must be willing and prepared to accept disappointment as part of what creates intimacy and authenticity in all of your most important connections.

Questions for Self-Reflection:

ϕ Do I allow others the space to communicate openly with me?

ϕ Am I open and honest in the way that I communicate with others?

LET'S GET R.E.A.L: ACCEPTING OUTCOMES

Accepting outcomes as they come sounds much simpler than it is, but I can't stress enough how important this concept is for your Emotional Mastery. You need to learn to accept outcomes, even if it means you are disappointed with them, and in truth, disappointment is a healthy part of any relationship. When we talked about assertive communication style, it's important to remember that being assertive isn't about getting what you want, but rather managing your own behavior without attempting to control others. Really, it's about being open, honest and authentic in your relationships, even if it means you have to accept an outcome that you were not expecting or is disappointing.

DISAPPOINTMENT IS ACTUALLY HEALTHY

When it comes to relationships, in order to truly accept the outcome of your assertive conversations, you need to be able to self-regulate and manage your anxiety. This oftentimes also means accepting disappointment, and in all honesty, I love talking about disappointment. I know it sounds funny, but the reason I do is because, growing up in a home with very loving parents, we didn't know how to disappoint each other. We sort of had this unwritten rule that, if you disappointed another person, it meant you didn't love them, and this was the idea I grew up with. As an adult, I carried forward this template, and for a long time, I believed that disappointment, love and intimacy could not coexist. Now, I know that to be the furthest thing from the truth, and I want you to know that disappointment is a natural and healthy experience in high-powered relationships, and you can allow yourself to be vulnerable and feel disappointed. Vulnerability and disappointment go hand in hand, and when you make the decision to be more open, honest and authentic in your relationships, you also make way for the experience of disappointment.

Vulnerability is critical to intimacy. In fact, intimacy is not possible without vulnerability, and true intimacy is not possible without disappointment, too. You have to understand that if you are going to truly deepen your relationships, you have to be willing to embrace this mindset that disappointment is healthy. You must be the one responsible for managing the disappointments that make way into your life. No one else is responsible for this, and sometimes, the reason you find yourself disappointed is simply because you predicted an outcome and it didn't go your way.

Questions for Self-Reflection.

φ How can I allow myself to be more vulnerable with the people that I love?

φ How do I approach disappointment?

STOP MAKING PREDICTIONS

In order to have a high-powered mindset, you need to be willing to stop making predictions about what is going to happen in your interactions and relationships with those in your life. It is so easy to fall into the trap of predicting how someone will react to information you are about to share, and I cannot stress enough how unhealthy this habit is. All those 'what if' scenarios just prepare you for a reality that may not be true, damaging your confidence and limiting your high-powered beliefs.

There were many times when I would think of asking my husband for something, but then wouldn't because of the prediction I had made that he would be angry or upset and deny my request. I thought my husband wouldn't understand, so I didn't even bother to tell him, and it was something I saw a lot of women in my practice experience too. This, however, isn't the thing to do. There is a saying that goes, "If you don't ask, then the answer is always no," and this applies here because you are not letting yourself accept the outcome. Instead, you are avoiding the outcome altogether, which does not help you to achieve your goals. When you ask a request of someone and they respond with, "I am so sorry, I can't do that for you," it's important to remind yourself that you are simply informing them of your preferences. In the end, it's up to them to decide if they will meet your requests, and you need to accept the outcome, and doing so gives you an amazing ability to navigate this with maturity and grade.

This component of the R.E.A.L. formula requires you to understand that it's your right and responsibility to express your preferences and needs, but it's not your right to control other people. You have absolutely no right to control or exercise any kind of manipulation. In fact, this is the furthest thing from an authentic connection. It's important to remember you are making a request, not a demand. It's not about being aggressive in the way you communicate in order to get what we want, but about being assertive in the way you communicate and accepting whatever the outcome is.

STOP TRYING TO CHANGE WHAT YOU CAN'T CONTROL

The very first thing acceptance requires is managing your own anxieties around the things you can't control. This is extremely important, and when it comes to taking radical responsibility for your own happiness, you need to be able to manage your anxiety to be able to communicate with confidence. You can't allow your preferences, anxieties and needs for control to get in the way of having authentic conversations. Anxiety is ultimately the focus on the things we can't control and is a natural part of our lives. This is my personal and professional definition of it, and the best antidote to anxiety is acceptance. In reality, the things you can't control are other people's choices, thoughts, feelings and outcomes. This is a very clear list and understanding this will really help you to accept all outcomes regardless of what they are. What I want for you more than anything else is to have an increased sense of awareness around your thoughts because it is your thoughts that drive your anxiety. If you are ruminating on other people's choices, thoughts, feelings and outcomes, the truth is, you are only really hurting yourself. You are not doing yourself and your ability to execute on Emotional Intelligence any good.

It is critical that you understand that when you decide to become more assertive in your relationships, you cannot control the outcome. In fact, I am going to push this even further and say it's others' rights and responsibilities to say no to you, and I can guarantee you that this acceptance of outcomes is the breeding ground for authenticity and intimacy in any relationship because there is a sense of equalness and understanding. Remember, communication is truly a two way street, and it's about both asking for your needs to be met and equally making space for the needs of others to be met, too. Once you have learned to accept any outcome, you can move on and learn to let go.

LET'S GET R.E.A.L: LETTING GO

Letting go is hands down the most powerful Emotional Mastery skill you can learn. In truth, you know you have never had control over outcomes to begin with, and while you can influence outcomes, you cannot actually control them. Understanding this crucial difference will make a massive difference in your life. Even if the outcome is something that really matters to you, like your child's entry into a school of their choice, your mother respecting a boundary you have put in place, or requesting more affection from your partner, the reality remains the same: you cannot control what happens on the other end of your requests and wants. So, how do we navigate through life with confidence when outcomes, particularly, the really important ones, are unpredictable? Well, you need to identify all of the things within your control, and then, identify all the things outside of your control. After you have identified these varying factors, you need to decide what you will take action on from the things within your control and commit to moving towards acceptance on the things you cannot control. While it may be difficult to accept things outside of your control, remember the importance of letting go. You will remain stuck if you do not. Just remember, the more you exercise habits that build your mental resilience, the more confidence you will experience in letting go and living a high-powered lifestyle.

THE ART OF HOLDING SPACE

Holding space was something I used a lot in therapy, and essentially, it's what allows for honest, non-judgmental exploration of self. I held space for my clients to explore and express their thoughts, feelings and choices and uncover what it is they needed to change in order to execute at their fullest potential. Now, I am asking you the same question. What are the things you need to do in order to execute at your fullest potential in your personal life and in your relationships? Just like I was holding space for my clients, it may be that holding space is what you need to do with yourself and with the important relationships in your life. Holding space takes a great deal of emotional maturity and Emotional Intelligence. I like to think of it as the ninja move in relationships. I also know it's one you can achieve.

You must let go of what you expect of others and hold space for what they actually need to express to you. It may not be an easy talk, but with practice, you will strengthen this muscle in your mindset and soon find yourself being able to truly engage in authentic and honest relationships with your loved ones.

Questions for Self-Reflection:

ϕ How can I hold space for the people I love?

ϕ How do I hold space for myself, my goals and my dreams?

In order to build better relationships, as women, we need to start by showing up differently in these relationships. We need to remember that we must make equal space for others and that communication truly is a two-way street. Remind yourself that disappointment is part of the process, and there is tremendous empowerment in taking radical responsibility for your own moods and the way you react to things that don't go your way. This all comes with mastering your emotions, which is the foundational pillar of success for relationship management. Once you are able to dial into your mindset and communication skills, you are able to set boundaries, say no and navigate your relationships without any shame. It's a combination of mindset, communication and relationship management that gets you out of the relationship trap and moves you towards building relationships that last.

CHAPTER SEVEN

LET'S GET TO THE C.A.S.E. — THE ASSERTIVENESS FRAMEWORK

"How can you take action if you don't have an actionable formula? There is a strong C.A.S.E for assertiveness."

"Why should I bother telling my husband how I feel if it won't change anything?"

"What is the point of asking for what I need if I know I won't get it?"

"Why would I be honest with my mother if I know she's just going to get upset with me?"

These are all thoughts I have had. In fact, I held the perspective that if things were not going my way and I couldn't control the outcome, there was no point in even having the conversation. Then, several years ago, I made a decision. I decided that I would change the trajectory of my relationships by communicating fearlessly with the people I love most, not in a manipulative effort to change them or the outcome, but so I could navigate my relationships with courage and integrity. I have since learned that assertive communication has *nothing* to do with getting what I want and *everything* to do with how I choose to show up in my relationships, and when my relationships are thriving, I am basically unstoppable. Taking action was what made it easy for me to elevate my relationships, and it's something you can do, too. So, I have created what I like to call the assertiveness blueprint, which include the four steps that you will need to execute assertive conversations and elevate your own relationships.

C.A.S.E., which stands for context, ask, specify, and embrace + let go, is the blueprint you can use again and again when you are ready to set boundaries and renegotiate your relationships. It's the framework that will help you have those difficult conversations when you want change in your relationships and allows you to plan these changes in advance so you can self-regulate when anxiety attempts to kill your confidence.

C.A.S.E: DEFINE THE CONTEXT BEFORE MAKING REQUESTS

Context is the very first step in having an assertive conversation. Before you move into making a request or having a difficult conversation, it is important that you define the context. Be clear, concise and to the point when you are communicating, and make sure not to give the other person a lecture. You don't want to start a conversation with, "You are so lazy and inconsiderate. You are always taking advantage of me. You don't care." This is a sure way to end the life of any healthy conversation. Clearly, if you were to say something like this to someone, you would be going "straight for the jugular" of the relationship. If you begin by accusing the other person of a negative personality trait, you invite them into a space of defensiveness, which essentially shuts down any further communication and you will not be able to actually action your request. What you want to do instead is engage in high-powered communication.

Start conversations by briefly defining the context, for example:

φ I have a lot to do before our guests arrive.

φ It has been quite some time since we have spent time together alone.

φ I noticed that the lawn has not been cut.

Communicating like this gives some context to the conversation you are wanting to have with this person and allows them to enter the conversation from a place of better understanding.

Someone who really inspired me to be clear in my communication and always provide context was my mentor. I met her in my mid-twenties. She was a clinical supervisor and the president of our association for couple and family therapy. In my eyes, she was the epitome of an Emotionally Intelligent Woman. She was an amazing clinician, inspiring leader, and the most wonderful mentor I've ever had. The way she held space for me to grow, explore and learn was incredible. I had so much respect for her personally and professionally. What I admired most about her was her ability to own her space, whether she was on a stage or casually having coffee with me. I had never met someone like that before who could be the exact same person when we were meeting for coffee as when she was giving a keynote. It was amazing how she could command a presence and give so much energy and passion to what she was saying. The way she showed up for every single one of our meetings, always in the same energy, in every context, was a magical skill that I think seamlessly helped her to manage her relationships and was something I knew I needed to learn to do myself.

It's important to keep in mind that the goal is still for you to make your request, and in order to not begin an argument when you do this, you want to provide a backdrop for your request by stating, in behavioral terms, the context of your request and where your request is coming from. You want the person you are communicating with to really understand your request, and if you take anything from this, it's that context is absolutely critical.

Questions for Self-Reflection:

- φ *How can I be more clear when communicating with others?*
- φ *How can I provide context for what I am feeling and thinking?*

C.A.S.E: WHEN ASKING, USE YOUR WORDS, NOT ACTIONS

Once you have given context, then you are ready to make your request, and there are a few principles that I want you to keep in mind when you are about to ask. The very first principle is to use words, not actions. You don't want to show your emotions, use facial expressions or be huffing and puffing. You don't want to slam things down or give the silent treatment. This would be being passive aggressive, and passive aggressive communication is manipulation. Instead, you want to always use your words and remain calm. Remember, this is all about emotional maturity and executing from a place of Emotional Intelligence.

Particularly when it comes to negotiating boundaries with your child, it's crucial that you remain calm and remind yourself that you are coming from a place of Emotional Intelligence. You don't want to come from a place of emotion because your child may react and fail to take in your words, and this goes for everyone you have a conversation with, too. Even if you are expressing how you feel and it's frustration, anger or hurt, it's important to try and use a calm, respectful and even tone. A simple statement saying you are frustrated is actually far more effective than yelling and snapping at someone.

TAKE RESPONSIBILITY FOR HOW YOU FEEL

Regardless of what you are feeling, it's up to you to take responsibility for your actions. Instead of saying, "You are making me overwhelmed. You are frustrating," try a different approach and say, "I am feeling overwhelmed. I am feeling frustrated." you will be surprised at the difference this makes. In conversations like these, it's also crucial that you avoid playing the blame game because, when you do so, you engage in passive aggressive and aggressive communication, which can hinder the relationship. Even though it may feel like you are going against your natural urges, take a breath (or five), adjust that Emotionally Intelligent crown of yours and take responsibility for your emotions *and* your actions.

When you are communicating your requests, it's far more effective to ask in terms of what you would like l rather than describe all the negative emotions that you are currently feeling and what you don't like. Instead of saying, "I get so angry when you are on your phone," try saying, "I want to feel close to you, could we watch a movie together?" Rather than focusing on the problem, you are communicating to the other person that you are interested in generating solutions and the concern you have is solvable, and this is a really powerful skill. This approach makes space for hope and a willingness to make changes. When you highlight the positive, or preferred, outcome and communicate to the other person that they are important to you and you value the relationship, it really helps to foster the intimacy you want.

DON'T PLAY THE VICTIM

When making requests, it is highly important that you don't play the victim. Playing the victim is incredibly manipulative, and it is an invitation for the other person to feel guilty. Take a deep breath, pause for a second and ask yourself this: are there moments in your relationships where you might want to invite the other person to feel guilty? We all do this, but it is a very ineffective way of deepening intimacy. The hope with playing the victim is that, essentially, the guilt the other person feels will force them to change and give into our request. That is really why we do it. That is why we try to invite guilt, and while it may work in the short run, in the long run, it will damage the relationship.

One of the things I want you to understand when it comes to relational dynamics is that certain things work, for example, manipulation might give you what you want in the moment, but they might also be highly ineffective and even problematic to the overall success of a relationship. When you use control, manipulation or guilt to get your needs met, what you are really doing is damaging the relationship, and it actually sets you up for failing when it comes to communication. Instead of approaching your request from your personal perspective, ask from a place where the other person best understands where you are coming from. Remember, be concise, be clear and be kind.

Questions for Self-Reflection:

φ *What am I feeling that I need to take responsibility for?*

C.A.S.E: SPECIFY WHAT YOU WANT

In terms of healthy, generative communication, specifying your preferred outcome goes a long way, and it is so important to be clear and concrete in your request. This is something I can't stress enough. Oftentimes, we are really general or broad with what it is we are looking for. Maybe, you want someone to love you more or want someone to show you they care, but, the truth is, generalizations like these actually make it really difficult to create any change in a relationship. So, it's important to communicate your preferences clearly and with specificity. Then, knowing you can't control the actual outcome, it's important to let go.

DECIDE WHAT YOU WANT

The first step in approaching a conversation with specificity is to know what you want and decide on what you want to communicate. I know it can be hard to be clear about your wants, needs and preferences, but the more specific you can be about your preferred outcome, the more fluid the conversation can be. That is one thing specificity really allows for: the conversation to just flow. Before even beginning the conversation with the other person, I want you to take some time to get really clear on what exactly you are asking for and how you will present your request. I want you to be concrete and specific, and trust me, this will take you a long way.

Questions for Self-Reflection:

φ *What is it that I want from my relationships?*

φ *What do I want more of in my life?*

φ *What do I want less of in my life?*

BE CLEAR, BE BRIEF

Along with specifying what it is you want, it's important to be clear and brief. I know that, once you get specific with what you want, it may seem like you have a list of things, but it really shouldn't take more than one to two sentences to communicate your request. Have you ever told someone that it feels like you are being lectured? Well, this is what happens when you do not approach the specifics of your request with clarity and brevity. So, instead of saying, "I would like you to do more around the house, all you do is sit around and watch TV all day," try saying "Could we take turns doing the dishes? I think it will give us more time to hang out after the kids go to bed. Would you be open to that?" Instead of expressing what you don't want, express what you do want. Be clear and concise, otherwise the other person may not have any actual clue of what it is you want. Placing your request in that specific and positive frame really allows the other person to know what it is you are looking for without damaging the relationship.

C.A.S.E: EMBRACE AND LET GO

Communicating fearlessly means managing your own emotions and behaviors without attempting to control others. It is being honest, open and authentic in your relationships, and often, it takes a lot of courage and confidence to ask for your needs while simultaneously accepting that we are not in control of the outcome. This is where having the courage to embrace the process of engaging with another person and being okay with discomfort and disappointment, and being let down or hurt comes in. This is really what the embrace section of C.A.S.E. is all about.

Embracing the negative experiences you can have and knowing that the outcomes are out of your control and that they have something to teach you is one of the most important components to developing a high-powered mindset. It's about embracing this discomfort fully and completely, and remembering that, when you make requests to others, you are simply informing them of your preferences. Now, to embrace is to understand that it's your right and responsibility to express your preferences, but it's not your right to control the other person, and this is the crucial piece that I want you to come to terms with. Embracing that we can't control or manipulate the other person's needs, preferences and opinions, particularly when they are different from your own, is not only a critical component of assertive communication, but also a critical component of having authentic relationships.

Communicating fearlessly, accepting and fully embracing disappointment in relationships is really hard, but ultimately, it's the backbone of all high-powered relationships. I know it's common to worry about other people's thoughts, feelings and actions, but the truth is, you only have control over your own. It's really what Emotional Mastery and being an Emotionally Intelligent Woman is about. It's getting a handle on managing your thoughts and emotions and driving your choices so that you can truly have a sense of personal agency over your life. With this, you truly are poised to execute on developing high-powered relationships.

Questions for Self-Reflection:

ɸ How can I better approach negative or difficult experiences?

ɸ What situations in my life am I trying to control?

ɸ What would happen if I allowed myself to let go?

Context is the very first step in our assertiveness framework, and it's important to make a request without starting an argument. Remember, when you ask, you need to use your words and not your actions, and be specific about what it is you want and what your preferences are. You must learn to be okay with not getting what you want and managing your emotions and behaviors without attempting to control others. Lastly, you must remember that we are all different, with different needs, opinions and preferences, and it's important to embrace these differences, especially when they vary from your own. All of these actions help you to have authentic relationships and allow you to thrive and become unstoppable.

I think back to ten years ago when I was struggling to navigate through my relationships and the truth is that, back then, I was so overwhelmed with my life that I would have shuddered at the idea of self-expansion. I really struggled to ask for my needs without replaying the conversation in my head for days. I struggled to ask for what I needed because I couldn't allow myself to even have that conversation if I felt the outcome wasn't going to go my way. I was so bogged down by my own emotions that I never dared dreaming of a bigger mission. I was feeling so personally stuck that I was becoming stagnant in my professional life. The turning point for me was recognizing that my personal relationships and, more accurately, my Emotional Intelligence skills were impacting my professional success, and this realization was a game changer. It was then that I knew I needed to shift my perspective and be the change I wanted to see in myself, not just for my own sake, but for my daughter, my husband and all the people I love. As I made the commitment to do my own deeper work, suddenly, there I was, stepping into the arena as a leader and owning two incredible businesses that serve people in powerful ways. Finally, it felt as though my personal life, my professional life and my mission were coming into alignment. And it felt amazing.

Over a decade ago, I decided I was going to get out of my own way so that I could experience success at a whole new level. I knew it was what I needed to become the Emotionally Intelligent Woman who had the capacity to embody the desires of her heart. The road to getting there started with taking a good, hard look at myself. Becoming aware of and owning all parts: good, bad and ugly. Nothing changes unless we do. Once we embrace this truth, the journey begins.

Part Three

Lead With Confidence

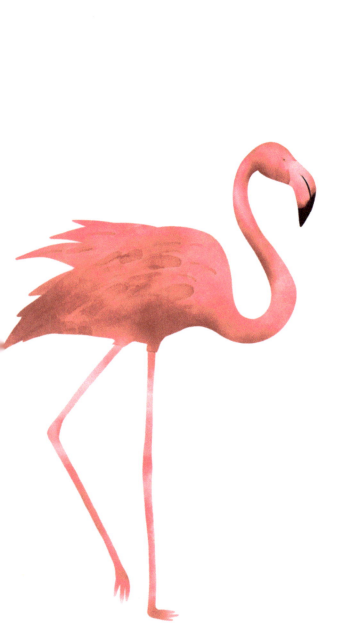

CHAPTER EIGHT

THE TOXIC TANGO OF RELATIONSHIP HABITS

*"I am not doing this toxic
dance with you anymore."*

I am about to get very vulnerable with you. I was a serial dater. It was through years of self-reflection and an increased awareness of my own patterns that I came to realize I wasn't only always in a relationship, but anxiously attached in my relationships. In all honesty, I hated being single and avoided it the best way I could, by jumping into relationship after relationship for most of my twenties. Then, I went through this period of time where I just swore off dating, and little did I know that it would be during this time that I would meet my husband. We met online, and this was during a time where online dating wasn't nearly as common as it is now. In fact, we were so embarrassed to say that we had met online that we actually lied about it for some time. On our first date, we went to a Cirque Du Soleil show, and I felt this instant connection to him. I am not going to say it was love at first sight (because now I know better), but he was very kind, respectful and so confident in who he was as an individual, that I found myself drawn to this new, healthy energy. We had these really great conversations. So, we kept seeing each other after that first date, and while it wasn't always easy along the way, we had shared dreams, values and hopes, the connection was there and we have been together ever since. While I was so happy to be with my soulmate, there were still pieces of the old me lingering around. I would still find that, despite the fact the relationship was going well, I would still experience anxiety in the relationship.

I remember distinctly this one time he went on a trip to New York to visit some family. Before he left, he had said to me, "Don't worry. We'll still talk every day," How did he know I was worried about that? Two days into his trip, and no phone call. At this point, I was making up all kinds of stories in my head about him and our relationship. I was super anxious, worked up and definitely catastrophizing. I had already gone to this awful place in my head, and in that moment, I told myself the relationship was over. My anxious attachment style was fully activated. If I perceived there to be a lack of safety, I would become distressed, even if nothing was actually happening. That trip my husband took to New York is when I first really felt the anxiety come up for me in the relationship with him, and he had done nothing to contribute to it. I might have had other partners that were not stable or secure, but he wasn't like that at all. It was all me. He finally did call while at The Cheesecake Factory with his cousin, but at that point I had already wound myself up pretty tight. He said he was going to have dinner and asked if he could call me later, but I was so anxious that I couldn't let him get off the phone. In that moment, I HAD to clarify: were we exclusive or was he seeing someone else? Yup. Anxious attachment rearing its ugly head again. I just needed to know. His response was, "Woah, can we have this conversation when I get back to Toronto?" Meanwhile, I was so worked up that I needed to know at that moment the "official status" of our relationship.

At this point in my life, I wasn't self-regulating the way I do now, and my husband still laughs about that phone call. I couldn't see that *he* was busy on that trip so we didn't talk as often. It didn't mean he didn't care. It just meant he was busy, and I had to remind myself not to personalize it. It took me time and experience to realize that just because my husband didn't do x, y, and z did not mean he was any less committed to me. We ended up having that conversation when he got back to Toronto, and I told him about my anxiety, but apparently he had already seen it. He was the first one to recognize the patterns. Was it really that obvious?!

In any relationship, it truly takes two to tango, and toxic relationship habits are a dance between the couple. The goal, however, is to tell your toxic relationship habits, "I am not doing this toxic dance with you anymore."

In my 20 years of working with people in a very intimate way, I have learned that people are experiencing more stress, pressure and overwhelm than ever before, and I think it's because we are feeling taxed on so many different levels. What I've noticed is that people are struggling more than ever to navigate their relationships, and relationship distress continues to be a powerful predictor of overall dissatisfaction in life and decreased mental health. One of the reasons I have written this book is because I have come to believe that many forms of self-help scratch the surface and can leave people feeling frustrated and hopeless. However, I am a believer that elevated relationships require that we each do our own work because relationships are strongest when we each take radical responsibility for our emotions and communication style. This is the magic formula, and in order to do the work, you need to look at *what* you need to work on, starting with your relationship thinking traps.

RELATIONSHIP THINKING TRAPS

Now, we have discussed thinking traps, but there are some thinking traps that are particular to relationships we need to go over, and they are mind reading, emotional reasoning, making demands and blaming. These particular thinking traps can really wreak havoc on your relationships, and it is important to recognize which thinking traps resonate with you in order to begin altering your mindset and replacing these toxic traps with high-powered thinking patterns and beliefs. In order to be the change you want to see, you first need to identify what needs changing, especially if it's at a subconscious level.

MIND READING...
BUT NOT IN THE SUPERHERO KIND OF WAY

Let's look again at that phone call I had with my husband while he was in New York. I was caught in this particular thinking trap where I was telling myself that he did not want to be with me because I had not spoken to him in two days. Reasonably, I would have noticed and told myself that he was busy, but in reality, I just gave into my negative thoughts and let them wreak havoc over me until he got back from his trip. I had this idea that I knew exactly what he was feeling and thinking without even talking to him. It's why I jumped at the opportunity to define the relationship even if the time wasn't right. Usually, when we do things like this, what we are doing is projecting our own stuff onto other people. It's believing with certainty that you know exactly what the other person is thinking and assuming they think the worst of you. It's mind reading, but in a completely inaccurate way. Instead of this 'mind reading' helping you in your relationship, what it does is actually hinder you because it's driven by low self-esteem, feelings of inadequacy, fear of rejection. It's a protective strategy you subconsciously use to keep yourself safe from criticism, but the reality is that it creates social anxiety and places you in constant worry about what others think about you, leaving you unable to authentically express yourself.

Questions for Self-Reflection:

ϕ Do I make assumptions about the relationships I have with others?

ϕ Do I project my insecurities into my relationships?

ϕ • Is it possible that I am unable to identify what others are thinking?

DON'T LET EMOTIONAL REASONING RUIN YOUR RELATIONSHIP

Have you ever felt jealous or suspicious in your relationship? Have you ever thought to yourself, "My partner must be cheating on me," even if you had no evidence to back it up? This is emotional reasoning, and it is a relationship toxin and thinking trap that will *really* wreak havoc on not just your relationships, but your mental state. It's this idea of taking your feelings or emotions and telling yourself they are absolutely true because you *feel* them to be true. Oftentimes, we fall into this relationship thinking trap when we have difficulty regulating our emotions and counteracting intense feelings with logic and rational thought, and that is what really drives this particular trap. It's developed by a focus on emotions in the absence of evidence-based reasoning, causing you to give your feelings a strong priority even if they are not reflective of reality. When you fall into the trap of emotional reasoning, what you are really falling into is elevated emotional dysregulation and poor decision-making. It pulls you out of touch with reality and makes it almost impossible for you to see facts, especially when other people are sharing those facts, making it really difficult to build authentic connections.

Questions for Self-Reflection:

- ϕ Do my negative thoughts and emotions determine my actions?

- ϕ How are my feelings informing the way that I am looking at the situation or the other person?

- ϕ What facts am I ignoring in order to reinforce what I am feeling?

WHEN MAKING DEMANDS, PUT YOURSELF IN THE OTHER PERSON'S SHOES

So, my husband and I don't celebrate Valentine's Day. Early on in our relationship, he told me that Valentine's Day wasn't a big deal to him and it was far more meaningful to express what we mean to one another in everyday moments. When he first shared this with me, I was instantly upset. I told myself that if he really loved me, he would get me roses, chocolates and all the other things that make Valentine's Day what it is. I remember asking myself, "If we don't celebrate Valentine's Day, does it mean we love each other less?" Once I calmed down and self-regulated, I actually thought about what he was saying without personalizing his perspective. I began asking myself different questions, like, "Do we have to celebrate our connection on a predefined day? Is the quality of our relationship defined by external standards and expectations?" Since then, I have massively shifted my perspective on the meaning of February 14th and Valentine's Day. I never demanded my husband get me roses, chocolates or anything else on Valentine's Day because I put myself in his shoes and realized I didn't want to demand of him something he had no desire of doing.

For over a decade now, we haven't celebrated Valentine's Day. There have been no roses, no chocolates, no hoopla. And that is okay. What my husband and I have found is our own language of connection, and no one else needs to understand it but us. For some, Valentine's Day is about the traditional expressions associated with love, but for others, it's entirely different. For my husband and I, it's enjoying the flexibility and seeing where the day takes us without expectations or demands. It has been something that has made the fabric of our relationship stronger, but for some people, Valentine's Day must be celebrated, and they end up making demands that actually begin to erode their connection.

Oftentimes, making demands causes communication and relationships to become rigid. What happens is you are making demands of other people based on what *you* think *they* should do. Instead of taking into consideration their preferences and putting yourself in their shoes, what you end up doing is fixating on *your* personal preferences and trying to push them onto someone else. It's driven by a need for control and keeping people close, but it actually has the opposite effect and causes people to pull away from you. Essentially, it's a lack of personal boundaries that you project onto others, which limits authentic and genuine intimacy. Now, sometimes, when you make demands, the people in your life may say yes, but they may not mean it or feel like they *can't* say no to you. In the end, what happens is you either push people away or those who do stay begin to find strategies to get around your demands. Then, the other person begins to lie or omit information so they don't have to deal with your demanding nature, which erodes the relationship as a whole on both sides.

Questions for Self-Reflection:

φ Am I empathetic to the needs of others?

φ Do I take into consideration what is important to the people I love?

φ Are my demands realistic or are they ultimately helping me align with a need for control?

STOP PLAYING THE BLAME GAME

Blaming is an obvious relationship toxin and thinking trap. It's when you tell other people that things are all their fault. It's the idea of blaming another person and seeing the other person as the source of a problem while ignoring or minimizing any part that you play in the conflict and expecting the other person to change or fix things. Now, this is a toxic thinking trap a lot of us have found ourselves in. A lot of us play the blame game in the hopes that we come out innocent. However, what a lot of us fail to recognize is how harmful this thinking trap is to our relationships.

Blaming is driven by a fear of rejection if you admit fault and an avoidance of taking responsibility for change. The truth is that, sometimes, you think you don't want to change. What you think you really want is for everyone around you to change because you think it would be easier, but that is not true. I think it's far more empowering when you take complete responsibility for your own change and for your own happiness. Playing the blame game actually leads to an inability to resolve conflict, and others are left feeling frustrated that the conflict is very one-sided. It creates distance in the most intimate relationships and definitely pushes people away. It may feel like it's providing a solution, but it's only short-term and ends up doing more damage than good.

Questions for Self-Reflection:

φ *Do I get in denial when blame is put on me?*

φ *How often do I blame others for situations, out loud or in my head?*

φ *How can I demonstrate my understanding? How will I be accountable for my part?*

IDENTIFY THE FOUR HORSEMEN, THEN CUT THEM OUT

You may or may not have heard of Dr. John Gottman, an American psychological researcher and clinician, but he is known for his work with couples, and in particular the four toxic habits he has studied that have the power to erode the intimacy levels of any relationship, especially romantic relationships. He calls them the four horsemen of the apocalypse, and I want you to reflect on yourself as I go through these four habits and really think about when you are falling into these traps.

Most people have toxic relationship habits, and criticism, contempt, defensiveness, and stonewalling are the most common toxic habits that we see in relationships that are really struggling. These are Dr. John Gottman's four horsemen, and they breed resentment, eat away at trust and create false senses of intimacy. Whether you realize it or not, these toxic habits are hindering you in more ways than you can imagine, and the first step to making that change in your mindset and behavior is by acknowledging the toxic habits you have.

CRITICISM HAS A TONE AND IT'S TIME YOU STOP USING IT

Criticism is one of the four horsemen, and it's an incredibly toxic relationship habit. It's also a really easy habit to notice because it has a harsh tone and often contains global statements. It's a way of speaking to another person that erodes their character and who they are. Here is the thing we often forget when we are engaged with criticism: we are always going to have differences in our relationships. You are always going to have differences in opinions and preferences, and it is actually healthy to disagree or have a complaint. In fact, it's natural. Now, what is not natural is criticism, and there is a huge difference between criticizing and disagreeing. A complaint simply indicates a specific situation with which you are unhappy, but a criticism is meant to make the other person feel bad about who they are.

I have a tendency to put tons of toppings on salads because, in my opinion, a salad is just not exciting without lots of toppings. It's my preference, but my husband and my daughter disagree with me on this. They have a different preference than me, and on multiple, separate occasions, they have told me, "I don't like when you put so many toppings on the salad," and that is perfectly okay. They have every right to communicate this with me, and I think they have the responsibility to communicate with me when I am doing something that they don't like because it allows us to deepen our connection. Criticism, on the other hand, is far more global. Imagine my husband and daughter telling me, "I hate toppings all over the salad. You don't know how to cook. You just don't care." Here, you can see how it goes from toppings on a salad to my ability to cook, to a harsh judgement about me as a person. Over time, this toxic habit can erode the relationship. Moreover, criticism is incredibly ineffective at resolving problems because it creates no space for generating solutions. What ends up happening is people get stuck in a gridlock when a relationship is peppered with ongoing criticism and it breaks down our self-confidence and, eventually, destroys the possibility of real connection.

Questions for Self-Reflection:

ϕ *How do I take feedback?*

ϕ *How do I deliver feedback? Does it ever come across as critical?*

LOOK IN THE MIRROR; ARE YOU DISPLAYING SIGNS OF CONTEMPT?

Contempt is the second horsemen, and in my opinion, it's a dangerous and toxic habit when it comes to relationships and whatever form it decides to show up in. Contempt is different from criticism in the sense that it's a more intense expression of criticism. It takes the content of criticism and adds some really powerful and really toxic nonverbal communication to it. In fact, what you are feeling in contempt is disgust towards the other person, making it virtually impossible to resolve conflict. This toxic habit can show up as sarcasm, cynicism, name calling, eye rolling, sneering, mockery, and even hostile humor. These are all examples of contempt, and as you read through them again, I want you to begin imagining how toxic these habits actually are. Let's look at how it can be taken one step further through belligerence, which is actually characterized by even more intense levels of anger and is actually a form of aggression that falls within the aggressive communication style. It basically adds an element of threat to contempt, which is extremely unhealthy and toxic to any kind of relationship.

Dr. John Gottman says couples who are contemptuous of each other are more likely to suffer from infectious illnesses than other people. He might have written this back in 1999, but the most current research, in terms of relationship distress and physical illness, continues to trend in this direction. The truth is that relationship distress does have an impact on not just our mental health, but our physical health, too. So, if you are dealing with contempt towards your partner, or anyone else for that matter, it's important to look in the mirror and recognize these toxic habits before they escalate and cost you the relationship. If your partner, or anyone else, has contempt towards you, this is the moment to communicate with confidence and clarity how this toxic habit is hindering your relationship.

Questions for Self-Reflection:

ɸ Do I often use sarcasm, mockery or hostile humor to communicate to others?

ɸ Do I feel disgust or loathing towards others or their behaviors?

DON'T BE SO DEFENSIVE

The third horseman is defensiveness, and even though there are times where it may be a natural response to feeling criticized or verbally attacked, it is actually proven that defensiveness is completely ineffective when it comes to resolving conflict as it blocks us from taking personal responsibility. When a person is criticizing or attacking someone else, or you are feeling attacked or attacking someone else, defensiveness really only tends to escalate conflict. Basically, it's a covert way of blaming the other person and invites the other person into a position of apologizing or backing down.

Sometimes, when a loved one is telling you something for your own good, something for your own growth, you don't even realize you are responding defensively. While, sometimes, you may feel like you are being verbally attacked by a loved one, it may just be the way you are perceiving it. This is why it's so important to be emotionally regulated. It allows you to approach your relationships with calm and confidence and stops you from responding to any unwanted communication with defensiveness.

Questions for Self-Reflection:

φ *Am I defensive of my actions and decisions when they are questioned?*

φ *Do I often feel as if I need to stand up for myself and prove why I am not in the wrong?*

STONEWALLING: THE RELATIONSHIP BURNOUT

Stonewalling is essentially relationship burnout. Often what we find in relationships that are experiencing quite a bit of distress is that people weave in and out of the first three toxic habits and feel burnt out in the relationship. Now, most relationships experience a state of distress simply because we have never been taught how to be in one. With so many of the women I have worked with, I have realized their issues stem from unresolved issues within their family of origin, and in particular, the mother-daughter relationship. It's very common, and it's something I have experienced myself.

Most parents in the earlier generations did not have access to this level of training in Emotional Intelligence, and it's important that we let our parents off the hook for not knowing any better. No one wants to believe that their mother or father is this awful person who didn't meet their needs. Our parents did the best they could with whatever was accessible, and what is accessible to us today is worlds apart from their reality. Today, we have so much research and so many resources, but our parents didn't even understand the importance of Emotional Intelligence. No one taught them any of this stuff, and this helps me to understand the relationship I have with my own mother. She was doing the best she could with the tools she had.

There was a time where every time I talked with my mom, there was underlying tension. This would trigger so much sadness and guilt in me, and it wasn't until I shifted my perspective that I realized I was stuck in an old narrative with her. I realized that I was waiting for her to be different or show up in a particular way. One day, when I got tired of waiting, I made the one decision I had control over. I decided that I would make the effort to improve the relationship. I decided to show up the way that I wanted to show up and stop waiting for others to "go first."

Most of us come from unhelpful, toxic and problematic relationship patterns, whether they are our own or the ones we have seen growing up. It's sad, but it's the truth, and given many of us were never taught how to communicate, we often shut down, become defensive and act childish. Instead of asking for what you need, you learn to play nice, people please or say nothing at all, and this is the biggest threat to your relationships and why the large majority of your relationships are far from being optimized. Silence is, in fact, the *silent* relationship killer and it can show up as stonewalling in your relationship. When you are not adding anything positive to the relationship or constantly making negative withdrawals, you are headed for relationship burnout. There is only so much negative, emotional arousal, constant negativity and toxicity, and distress and conflict a relationship can take, and that is what stonewalling actually is. So, here is the toxic cycle that I am talking about. We have criticism and contempt, which in abundance leads to defensiveness, which continues to cycle through criticism and contempt until you eventually move into stonewalling, shutting down emotionally and tuning the other person out.

Now, stonewalling doesn't just show up in romantic or intimate relationships, but it really addresses all kinds of relationships, and I am going to give you an example that we can draw from a parent-child relationship. Let's say, for example, every time my daughter brings home an assignment from school, she shows me her grades and I criticize her lack of effort. I call her lazy and tell her she does not care about her future. This is criticism, and every time she brings home a grade from school that I am not happy with, what is naturally going to happen is she's going to defend herself. She's going to say things like, "Oh, the teacher doesn't know what she's doing. It's too loud at home to study," and she's going to make up all these excuses for the fact that I am criticizing her through her grades. Then, let's say I up the ante on my arguments and use more contempt. She's going to come back with more defensiveness until she reaches relationship burnout and throws on her headphones, cranks the music and stonewalls me whenever I try speaking to her about school. This is where the four horsemen can take you, and your relationships can reach a stalemate. So, if you are not communicating assertively, confronting issues and dealing with them as they come in a calm and collected manner, your relationships can truly reach that stalemate where the other person is completely withdrawn and provide very little or no verbal feedback that they are actually listening to us.

Questions for Self-Reflection:

φ Do I become easily irritated when things in my relationships don't go my way?

φ Do I pretend not to hear others' questions or comments and try to ignore them?

REDEFINING AND RENEGOTIATING YOUR RELATIONSHIPS

In order to cut out the four horsemen and all toxic relationship thinking traps, you must be willing to be self-reflective, do your own work and actually look at when and how it is that you fall into these particular habits and patterns. Redefining and renegotiating your relationships is really hard work, but it's also one of the most rewarding things you can do for your relationships. Once you truly learn to lean into the discomfort that is required to transform your relationships, you are ready to take the necessary steps to create high-powered, authentic relationships and lead with confidence. To combat relationship distress, you need to be self-reflective and self-aware and do the work and be the change you wish to see.

My husband and I still laugh about that phone call when he was in New York, and I value how much I have grown since then. The same goes with my mother. I value our relationship now more than ever before, and it all started when I paid attention to my toxic relationship habits and stopped dancing with them. It was learning that in every relationship, there are healthy habits and unhealthy habits, there is a need for both separateness and togetherness, and the importance of leading with confidence so that I can become an Emotionally Intelligent Woman and watch my relationships flourish.

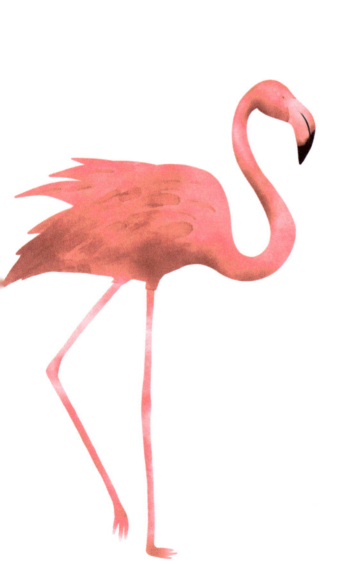

CHAPTER NINE

TOGETHERNESS

"Together, but separate."

If you grew up in Toronto in the 90s, you knew Fluid nightclub was the place to be every Thursday. Mary J. Blige, Biggie Smalls, and Boys II Men, all pumping through the speakers. Hoop earrings, flared jeans and acrylic nails were all the rage. I was there, ready to have a good time, and with my regular entourage: my girlfriends and our respective boyfriends. Then, like clockwork, my boyfriend and I got into an argument. I can't remember all the details, but I am certain it was about something inconsequential. He left the club, and my heart sank. No longer was I in the Thursday night spirit. Instead, I just wanted to go home and hide away under the covers, hoping he had come back around. It was my girlfriend that pulled me out of my funk. She turned to me, drink in one hand, and said, "He has to love all of you, good, bad and ugly. If he can't accept all of you, he's not worth it." Casually, she turned away and just kept dancing.

We couldn't have been more than 19 years old at the time, and I couldn't make sense of how my friend and I could have such different perspectives. I was flooded with panic at the fact my boyfriend had just left and she was suggesting that I own my worth, cut my losses and carry on. At the time, I had no idea what she meant. As fate would have it, about a decade (and a lifetime) later, I would become almost exclusively focused on understanding the science of relationships. I would learn that the reason I had such a visceral reaction to the possibility of rejection while my girlfriend effortlessly maintained her cool came down to attachment style. I was anxiously attached and my friend was securely attached. I pursued more connections when I was anxious. On the other hand, my friend was able to hold her own sense of confidence in her relationships. This difference in attachment style made a world of difference in how we saw ourselves and how we navigated our relationships.

One of the most valuable and magical concepts I've learned is that I can transform my early attachment patterns and regain control of my life, and so can you. It's this idea of "together, but separate" and "separate, but together," and it all has to do with attachment styles. When you feel safely and securely attached, when you have that secure base, you actually have a far greater propensity to behave and think independently and be more confident, and it all comes with looking at your attachment style and changing what needs to be changed. There is quite a bit of research and literature on attachment styles, and some of these concepts may be somewhat familiar to you, but what you are really going to be looking at are the three primary attachment styles: secure attachment, anxious attachment and avoidant attachment. Now, you may fall anywhere along the continuum of these attachment styles, so it's important to reflect and look at your family of origin. For many people, myself included, family origin work is not easy, but I am committed to continuing to be open and vulnerable with you by sharing my experiences. Remember, you and I are on the exact same journey. I may be a few steps ahead, but I continue to do this work every day.

ATTACHMENT AND ASSERTIVENESS GO HAND IN HAND, AND IT STARTS WITH YOUR FAMILY OF ORIGIN

While our Emotional Mastery has a lot to do with our ability to communicate fearlessly in specific situations, our overall ability and willingness to communicate assertively is actually largely influenced by our past relationship templates, especially those handed down by our primary caregivers. Now, the emotional bond you have with another person is called attachment, and your early attachment relationships are essentially what provide the template for understanding and interacting in future relationships. This template informs how you see yourself, how you see others, and ultimately, how you manage your emotions and share with others. Attachment can be a deeply nuanced and complex concept, which is why I wanted to make sure that you had a solid framework of emotion management and communication styles before I presented to you how to fully understand attachment styles. Ultimately, these templates will inform your mindset and influence your core beliefs about yourself and others.

When you look at your early relationships and family of origin, what you are looking at are the feelings, needs, desires and opinions you believe are acceptable to acknowledge and express. Typically, those "rules" around what feelings are okay to express and which ones are not okay are communicated covertly, or indirectly. My mother never came right out and told me, "Listen, Shyamala, it's not okay for girls to get angry. You are not allowed to express anger." I just picked up that template because of unwritten rules and from watching how my mother behaved within our family of origin. A keen awareness of your attachment style, core beliefs and communication template are actually what empower you and allow you to make better choices for yourself, which will unlock your ability to make choices about how you want to show up in your relationships.

LOOKING THROUGH THE ATTACHMENT LENS

In therapy, we often refer to attachment as a lens. Think of it like a pair of glasses that clinicians put on to view people and how they navigate their relationships. Now, attachment theory, which is where we get our attachment lens from, was originally introduced by Dr. John Bowlby in 1958, and what he suggested was that humans have an innate physiological need to form an emotional bond with caregivers, and having a strong bond is critical to a healthy development. Bowlby observed the distress patterns of institutionalized infants that were separated from their parents, and the very first stage of attachment distress Bowlby noticed was that the children protested the separation and were visibly upset. Then, he noticed that the children were beginning to express despair and were withdrawing. The final stage he noticed was that the children were expressing detachment and were becoming non-responsive. What Bowlby witnessed was children's behaviors becoming both progressively and predictably distressed after being separated from their parents, and it was through this study and Bowlby's observations that we began to understand the impact our early relationships have on us. From this attachment lens, what we have come to understand is that there are four particular elements of attachment that children naturally develop.

THE ELEMENTS OF ATTACHMENT

The four particular elements of attachment are proximity maintenance, secure base, safe haven, and separation distress, which develop naturally in children and continue to exist on an experiential level when we become adults even though we play them out differently in our adult relationships. These four elements are what essentially provide the template to your adult relationships, and in particular, your most intimate adult relationships. Now, when I say most intimate adult relationships, I don't simply mean romantic relationships, in any kind of relationship. Understanding these elements in children as well as in adults can help you to become aware of them so that you can actually work with them instead of having them control you.

PROXIMITY MAINTENANCE

The very first element of attachment is proximity maintenance. I know it's a bit of a fancy term, but what it simply means is a desire to be close to attachment figures and maintain physical closeness. We all have this innate desire to be close to the people in our lives that represent security and safety, and proximity maintenance is a very, natural, normal and healthy desire. As children, we have a natural desire to be close to our caregivers, and we see this desire continue into adulthood with attachment figures like our partners, our own children and other close loved ones. In adult relationships, proximity maintenance is simply wanting to spend time with and be close to another person. It may simply be wanting to hang out on the couch, in the same room, or have dinner with another person. Essentially, it's the idea of wanting to be physically close and spend time with someone else.

Questions for Self-Reflection:

 φ Do I put aside doing things for myself to spend time with my loved ones?

SECURE BASE

The second element of attachment is a secure base, and I quite like this one. It's the idea that the caregiver or attachment figure plays the role of a safe and secure base from which the child can explore the larger world. Research tells us that, when we feel safely and securely attached, we have a greater propensity for independence and are more confident. Interestingly, two seemingly opposite concepts come together to really help us optimize our lives and our relationships, and we can see this vividly in toddlers on their first day at school. Before entering the classroom, as the toddler walks away from a parent, the toddler looks back to make sure the parent is still there. This is because, as the toddler physically separates his or herself from the parent, all he or she needs to do is look back and take in the information that the parent is still there and can carry on.

As adults, having a secure base in our relationships can make us feel more confident. Having a secure base gives you more courage and you are more willing to take risks. You feel like you can accomplish anything, and the truth is it's because you feel valued and cherished by another person, which allows you to be more independent. When you are securely attached, you are more likely to do the things that may have really scared you before because you are more willing to try new things. You put yourself outside of your comfort zones because you know you have a secure base you can come back to.

Questions for Self-Reflection:

φ How do I feel when I take risks and step out of my comfort zone??

φ Do I feel a sense of security in my relationships?

SAFE HAVEN

The next element of attachment is safe haven, which is this idea that we can continue that process of independence and actually begin to tolerate separateness. What many people do not realize is that separateness is actually a healthy part of attachment, and going back to the toddler example, this is where that toddler returns to the caregiver for physical comfort, like a hug or a kiss, when he or she feels threatened or scared. I like to think of it almost like a lighthouse, a place that I know I can come back to and feel safe and cared for if I have had a hard day or when the world might feel a bit scary or challenging. Similarly to secure base, the idea of having a safe haven in an adult relationship is like the idea of coming home after a long day. It's knowing you can count on support and encouragement from another person, even if it's not verbally expressed. It's knowing they believe in you and believe you can do this.

This safe haven can exist in romantic relationships, but it can also exist in friendships and the relationship between a parent and an adult child.

Questions for Self-Reflection:

> ɸ How comfortable do I feel being apart from the people I love most?

SEPARATION DISTRESS

The final element of attachment is separation distress. It's the emotional distress expressed by children when they are separated from their parents or caregivers, and to continue with the toddler example, if you have ever seen a toddler have a difficult first day of school experience, you have typically seen the distress that comes over him or her. This is separation distress; it's normal and can be a healthy developmental stage for children to go through. Similarly, slightly evolved patterns of protest, despair and detachment can be observed in adult relationships when faced by threats. You can see separation distress in adults when they become upset and tear up when saying goodbye to a loved one before a long trip or if they are ill, and you see this quite a bit in friendships and in couples as well. It's an element of attachment you want to be aware of when those distress patterns carry on for extended periods of time because they can lead to relationship distress.

Questions for Self-Reflection:

> ɸ Do I become anxious and distressed when separated for too long from my loved ones?

IDENTIFYING YOUR ATTACHMENT STYLE

From attachment theory and the elements of attachment, we have now developed attachment styles, and this is probably a concept you have already heard about, especially as there is increasing research, literature and evidence-based models of working with people based on their attachment styles. Originally, attachment styles were identified by developmental psychologist Dr. Mary Ainsworth in 1979 when she took John Bowlby's work a step further and observed the attachment relationships between caregivers and their one-year-old children. In this study, the children were systematically separated and reunited with their mothers, and this is where Ainsworth identified the three overarching primary attachment styles, which are secure attachment, anxious attachment and avoidant attachment. Clinical psychologist and couples' therapist Dr. Sue Johnson has also helped to take these concepts a step further and put them into a usable, evidence-based framework that allows couples to develop healthier and more secure attachment styles based on their historical relationship patterns.

SECURE ATTACHMENT

Secure attachment is the attachment style that helps us build high-powered, elevated relationships. It helps us lead with confidence and gives us the ability to be close and trusting of others while simultaneously feeling empowered towards independence and separateness. Developing a secure attachment style is one of the strongest predictors of relationship satisfaction as well as overall satisfaction in life.

Now, you may be asking yourself what secure attachment style looks like in adults, and the answer is it's everything we have been covering. With a secure attachment style, you are self-aware, emotionally regulated, and are able to remain present and empathetic in your relationships. It's the ability to be aware, navigate and trust other people and allow people to get close to you and believing that relationships can be healthy and your needs can be met.

Secure attachment style is balancing the art of togetherness and separateness in your relationships, and when this happens, it's truly a beautiful thing. With a secure attachment style, you can enjoy time to yourself *and* time with others. You will experience yourself as confident, capable and full of courage, ready to take risks and take on the world, and you will experience your relationships as safe and they will feel connected and fulfilling to you. Essentially, you will experience the world as exciting and full of opportunities.

Questions for Self-Reflection:

φ Do I enjoy spending time with loved ones as well as having time to myself?

φ Am I aware of my emotions?

ANXIOUS ATTACHMENT

Anxious attachment style is characterized by the intense distress felt when separated from a loved one. It's finding it difficult to soothe, calm down or feel safe again, sometimes even when you are reunited with that loved one. With an anxious attachment style, you tend to be clingy and feel overwhelmed, and if you don't work through your anxious attachment, it can lead to feelings of sadness, intense loneliness, and of course, anxiety. Oftentimes, this is the style that is expressed with anger and bitterness and is made obvious through demands. Now, I want you to be really self-reflective here and think about those times and relationships where you might have fallen into the anxious attachment style. You might have experienced clinginess in the relationship, a need to constantly be close to the other person and anxiety about being separated from this person. Anxious attachment is like separation distress 2.0. It's a really intense feeling of separation, stress and overwhelm. It's having difficulty separating thoughts and feelings, and that is why it's critical to learn how to make the distinction between the two, so you don't fall into emotional reasoning. If you are anxiously attached, it's almost impossible to be assertive or communicate with confidence.

With an anxious attachment style, you might experience yourself as insecure at times, and I would say probably insecure most times when it comes to your personal and maybe even your professional relationships. You might experience your relationships as unsettling and may even become anxious when you are relating to others. You experience the world as scary and unpredictable, and there is almost a sense of being on the edge most of the time. If you are struggling with an anxious attachment style, you might find yourself gravitating towards a negative mindset, and when you are overwhelmed or distressed, chances are, you are going to fall deeper into that negative thinking. This style really creates a vicious cycle because you probably struggle with emotional regulation. When you feel anxious, it really eats away at your confidence, which makes it really difficult to make decisions, say no, set boundaries and actually practice assertiveness in your relationships.

Questions for Self-Reflection:

ɸ *Do I rely on others' approval to feel good about myself?*

ɸ *Do I worry about my loved ones when I am not with them?*

AVOIDANT ATTACHMENT

Avoidant attachment is similar in some ways to anxious attachment—although avoidant attachment goes in the opposite direction. When you are struggling with an avoidant attachment style, there is very little distress when you are separated from a caregiver or loved one. However, don't let this fool you. Separation distress is normal, and it's actually what pulls you back into a healthy attachment, but people with an avoidant attachment style typically appear distant and have difficulty connecting with loved ones. Now, if you don't address this and don't work on it, avoidant attachment can actually lead to feelings of sadness and loneliness because you are constantly pulling away and creating too much space in your relationships. It can even, eventually, lead you to an overwhelming sense of helplessness around how to properly navigate your relationships and you may end up expressing coolness or frustration to mask the vulnerability of feeling helpless. Again, I want you to be very self-reflective here and see what behavioral characteristics of an avoidant attachment style you may exhibit so you can work through it. With avoidant attachment style, there is discomfort with emotional closeness and even physical closeness. There is a fear of really being seen and showing who you are, so you may feel content just interacting on a surface level. With an avoidant attachment style, you may even be unaware of your thoughts and feelings because you may be highly detached from your emotions.

This attachment style shows up during conflict or stress, with the belief that it's better to let things go than to talk about emotions or have conversations about them within the relationship. It's not that these things aren't important, but it's a way of avoiding them. If you are struggling with an avoidant attachment style, you may see yourself as a lone wolf because you find close, emotional connections intimidating, and quite frankly, experience your relationships as empty or unsatisfying. So, you compartmentalize in order to create and keep distance. Like the anxious attachment style, during times of stress, if you have an avoidant attachment style, you might gravitate towards negative thoughts and beliefs and really struggle with mastering your emotions. You might struggle with identifying your emotions, which may make you even more detached, but it's making room to deal with the discomfort of opening up to others and really finding how you *feel* that can open you up to the possibility of exhibiting characteristics of a secure attachment style.

Questions for Self-Reflection:

ϕ Do I feel suffocated in relationships, particularly with romantic partners?

ϕ Do people tell me I am aloof or distant in several different relationships?

DON'T PROJECT YOUR ATTACHMENT STYLE ONTO OTHERS

The primary attachment style tends to continue into adulthood and show up in most of your relationships. If you gravitate or operate out of one particular attachment style, you may think that everyone operates that way. If you are anxiously attached, you may think everyone is anxiously attached. If you are avoidantly attached, you may think everyone is avoidant in their relationships. With this, what ends up happening is that you may be projecting your own attachment style onto others. If these attachment patterns are unhealthy, they may be the culprits of our relationship distress.

Understanding your attachment style is critical, and it's truly the first step in fostering high-powered relationships. Therefore, you need to have a keen awareness of your particular attachment style so that you really begin that work. Do not allow your attachment style, whether anxious or avoidant, to hinder you and your relationships. Instead, aim to develop a secure attachment style and understand that self-awareness around attachment, communication and emotions are what are going to allow you to make better choices for yourself and show up powerfully in your relationships. Understand that separateness is a healthy part of attachment. Separateness, along with, togetherness are both required for the high-powered relationships you want to foster.

Esther Perel is a psychotherapist and another one of my mentors, and while I have never had the opportunity to meet her in person, she has mentored me through her work and contributions to the field, especially for couples therapy. She is well-known for couples therapy, and she describes the importance of both togetherness and separateness beautifully when she says, "Love rests on two pillars, surrender and autonomy. Our need for togetherness exists alongside our need for separateness." From my experience, I can confidently tell you that this couldn't be truer. Maybe, if someone would have told me about attachment styles after my argument with that boyfriend I had at Fluid nightclub, I could have started my journey of becoming securely attached earlier. Today, I am grateful that somewhere along the way, I decided to do the work to transform my attachment style, for me, for my daughter, for my husband, and for all of my relationships. The most beautiful and inspiring relationships I have ever seen are two people navigating the space between themselves with love, respect, and ease, through togetherness and separateness.

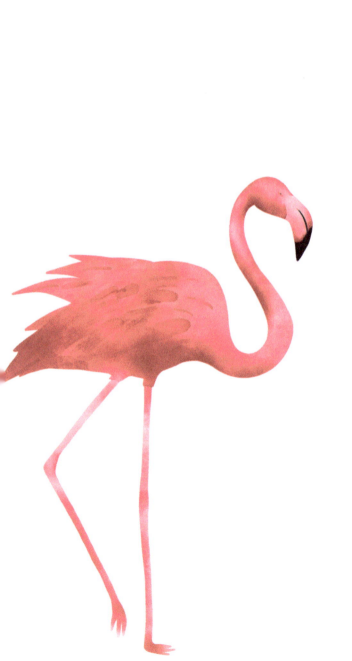

CHAPTER TEN

SEPARATENESS

"Separate, but together."

As you may recall from the story of my nightclubbing days, I used to have an anxious attachment style, which is something that is very common for women. I used to look for a sense of belonging in intimate relationships and lose myself once the relationship was over. I didn't know how to be in a relationship and be independent at the same time. I was constantly seeking connection to soothe my own anxieties and would feel even more anxiety when I was separated from my partner. Sometimes, I would even feel anxious when we were together, and even then, I felt like I never had enough togetherness.

Now, things are different, and I feel more securely attached in all of my relationships. I now have the ability to be deeply connected to my loved ones while simultaneously being able to maintain my sense of independence. Now, I can feel close in relationships without losing myself in them, and that is what authentic connection is about. It's talking with someone and feeling this great energy, but knowing where to find yourself in it. Essentially, it's recognizing that you are your best self when you feel safely and securely attached, have that secure base, and thus, have far greater propensity to behave and think independently and be more confident. In fact, in order to regain control of your life and fully execute on your mission of becoming an Emotionally Intelligent Woman and succeeding at everything you wish to succeed in, it's necessary to transform your early attachment patterns and relationship style.

DIFFERENTIATION

One of the things that I have noticed many people struggle with, and I struggled with too, was maintaining a sense of self and individuality when getting really close to someone in a relationship. However, what I know about high-powered relationships is that, essentially, they allow us to navigate togetherness and separateness, and this is ultimately the mark of a healthy relationship. Attachment theory assumes we are emotionally interconnected with one another. While attachment speaks to our human need for connection and closeness with others, differentiation is what allows us to balance our individuality and connection in these relationships. It's the ability to navigate life from a place of authenticity and integrity rather than from a place of projected or false self. We know that we sometimes project a false self to avoid conflict or placate others, but doing so is actually a strong predictor of relationship distress and is actually a cycle that keeps conflict going. However, when you operate from a differentiated self, you are actually able to identify your thoughts and feelings and respond from a place of emotional maturity, which is essentially what emotional mastery and fearless communication are all about. Differentiation is truly what I would consider the epitome of a high-powered relationship. It's learning to navigate your relationships from that place of differentiation, and the truth is that this skill is something you need to learn, especially if you didn't learn it with your family of origin. It's possible that your family of origin was structured from a place of low-level differentiation, and it's necessary to understand the different levels of differentiation and the impacts they can have on you and your relationships.

LOW-LEVEL DIFFERENTIATION

The most common relationship and differentiation template we see is what is called low-level differentiation. Low-level differentiation is essentially losing your sense of self and individuality when in a relationship. When there is low-level differentiation in relationships, assertiveness is not actually acceptable. It's not okay to be direct, open or honest and it's not acceptable to express thoughts or make choices that are not in line with the norms, rules or identities this relationship has adopted. Families with a low-level of differentiation tend to operate as a unit and put pressure on any family member that attempts to step out of line or does not want to maintain the status quo. You might have heard of the term emotional fusion, and this is simply the idea of too much closeness, which is what we see in relationships with low-levels of differentiation. It's the idea that, if I feel sad, then you feel sad. If I am upset, then you are upset. It's taking on other people's stuff as your own. Yet, sometimes, low-levels of differentiation are more subtle and not always as obvious as you might think. Parents with low-levels of differentiation, for example, might become triggered or flooded with emotions in situations where their child is upset or in distress. These parents will take on their child's emotions as their own, and what happens here is this reaction actually gets in the way and inhibits the parents' ability to respond well to their child's needs, which isn't what you want in any relationship. It is certainly not a healthy pattern or the ideal template for high-powered relationships.

Questions for Self-Reflection:

ϕ What emotions was I able to freely express in my family of origin?

ϕ Which emotions was I unable to express?

HIGH-LEVEL DIFFERENTIATION

With high-level differentiation, you are able to think with more clarity, take responsibility for your feelings and choices and make room for others to do the same. This is where you can communicate fearlessly and be able to self soothe your own anxieties. It's also where you can meet the needs of your loved ones, and I truly do believe that. When you have high-levels of differentiation, you allow yourself to show up as your best self in all of your relationships. A highly differentiated individual is able to maintain their sense of self and individuality while enjoying closeness and intimacy in a relationship.

Going back to the parent-child relationship example, when parents are highly differentiated, they are able to keep their emotions separate from their child's. They have the ability to remain calm, and therefore, have the ability to choose how they respond to their child's needs. Now, I think there is a misconception that the closer you are in your relationships, the healthier those relationships are. The truth is, there needs to be some space and distance in your relationships so that you can show up well, particularly when there is distress. high-level differentiation, especially in families, allows for the acceptance of a wide range of feelings, thoughts, needs, and desires, and conflicting feelings, thoughts, needs, and desires don't necessarily create a sense of anxiety or overwhelm within that family system. Instead, family members with high-levels of differentiation tend to engage with one another from a place of calm and mutual respect, and a family member can express a difference of opinions, and sometimes, even values, with room for acceptance, openness and disagreement, which is important for the authenticity and connection of the relationship.

CONNECTING DIFFERENTIATION WITH ASSERTIVENESS AND ATTACHMENT STYLE

As you know by now, assertiveness is really important in high-powered, elevated relationships, and if you are going to have these amazing relationships and lead with confidence in everything you do, you need to learn to be direct, honest and open. Differentiation allows for a greater capacity for all of the elements that foster great relationships. Your ability to communicate fearlessly, or be assertive, in essence, is a manifestation of differentiation. When you are highly differentiated, you are able to maintain your sense of self in the midst of your relationships and you are better equipped and able to manage the discomfort that sometimes comes with having difficult conversations.

Differentiation also intersects with attachment style, so it's critical that we understand how these concepts are correlated. I want you to look for yourself within these ideas and identify where you fall into these particular equations. If you have an anxious attachment style, you would have low-level differentiation and have very little separateness in your relationships and a very high need for closeness. You might have a very low sense of self and would want to be together with the person all the time. If you have an avoidant attachment style, you will also have low-level differentiation and have a very low sense of self, but be avoidant of emotional closeness or togetherness, creating distance and separateness in your relationships.

Now, if you are securely attached, you would typically have high-levels of differentiation and are able to maintain your sense of self and sense of separateness while in relationships and stay in the middle of the continuum. Ultimately, differentiation is a continuum. On the far left and right sides, you have low-level differentiation where you feel your sense of self being eclipsed, covered, consumed or overwhelmed by others and you get lost in your relationships or you are just completely avoidant. Then, in the middle, you have high-level differentiation where you feel able to express your thoughts, feelings, needs and desires despite the fact that they might be different form the people you are in a relationship with and you are able to maintain a sense of self and your individuality while maintaining also a sense of togetherness or closeness. Now, nobody can achieve this transformation overnight. In fact, you can move in and out of these particular elements in your relationships at any given moment, but with practice, it gets easier, even if it will always be a work in progress. You are not alone in this.

In full transparency, I continue to navigate these elements every day. It's perfectly normal in times of stress to move towards an anxious or avoidant attachment style, but it's important to come back to your secure base. Remember, you want to consistently land in the middle, in that zone that leaves you feeling safely and securely attached. Emotional Mastery leads to fearless communication, which intersects with elevated relationships: this is how high-powered relationships are built. This is how you lead with confidence in *all* of your relationships. When you are highly differentiated, it means you truly have the ability to practice assertiveness from a place that is emotionally neutral, and you are able to communicate with confidence, regulate emotion and engage in your relationships in a healthy way. The more you combine these elements and practice them as a system for success, the better able you are to have high-powered relationships and become the Emotionally Intelligent Woman I know you can be.

There was a particular woman I worked with who had been in therapy for 15 years prior to working with me, and I remember how well I could relate to her struggles. She would get in her own way and in her own head, and whenever a conversation frayed or went even a little sideways, she would become aggressive and things would escalate very quickly. When I met her, she had no idea how to manage any of it, let alone find the confidence and connection she longed for. When we started our work together, she was ready to leave her husband and cut off her sister. By the end of our work together, not only did she reconnect deeply with her husband and reconcile with her sister, she also decided to scale and grow her own business. She was leading herself, and her life, with confidence. With an increased sense of personal power and personal agency in her life, she found herself reaching for goals she would have never imagined in the past. She transformed her old patterns of thinking, communicating and relating, and in doing so, she's had the deep privilege of meeting the most powerful version of herself: her Emotionally Intelligent Self.

I live for these sorts of transformations because committing to all of these practices has really transformed me from a woman who admired assertiveness and confidence in others to being able to *be* assertive and confident herself. Now, I am able to show up for myself as well as for the people in my life that matter most. I am able to contribute fully to my mission and serve from a place of power and integrity.

Ten years ago, I was a completely different person, and I knew I wanted to share my story in some capacity, but my story ten years ago wasn't what it is today. Now, I host a podcast, *Confessions of an Ex-Therapist*, and it's something I had always dreamed of doing but never had the confidence to do before. I knew I wanted to demystify this idea that therapists have everything together and that their life and relationships must be perfect. I knew I wanted to help normalize others' experiences by telling my own story and help other women become their Emotionally Intelligent Self, living high-powered lives. Through my experiences, I was able to learn the importance of "together, but separate" and "separate, but together," and that separateness is recognizing that I am me and you are you. I was able to learn to communicate fearlessly, and mostly, be the change that I wanted to see in myself. It's amazing what has happened in my life and in my relationships because of these concepts, and it's the reason why I've written this book now. It's the reason I knew I wanted to share all of this with you and help you become this high-powered woman with a better understanding of herself and what she wants to achieve in life and in her relationships. I have no doubt in my mind that, if you commit to showing up as your best self, you will become your best self. While we are nearing the end of our journey together in this book, your journey of becoming is only just beginning.

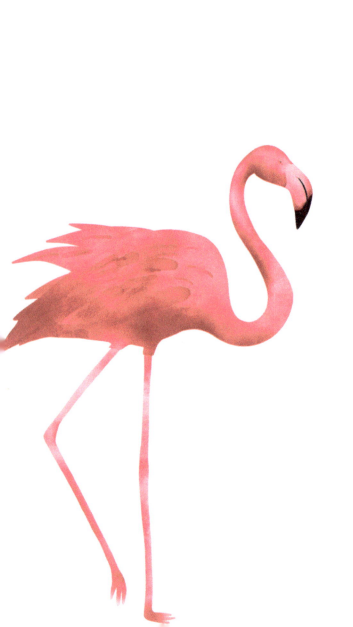

CHAPTER ELEVEN

BUILD YOUR BLUEPRINT FOR EMOTIONAL INTELLIGENCE

"Mummy, I think I should be a guest on your podcast," my daughter told me in the car as we were on our way home from school.

After I released the first episode of my podcast with a guest speaker, my daughter and I listened to it as I drove her to school. The interview was with a brilliant woman who is a naturopathic doctor and created an out-of-the-box way of delivering community healthcare, and I guess it must have stayed with her because, when I picked her up from school, she told me she wanted to be a guest on the podcast. She told me, "I can do that," and it was one of those moments I'll never forget.

"Tell me more", I asked. She said, "You talk about emotions, and I can talk about the effects a parent's stress can have on the child." In that moment, I recognized that, at 11 years old, my daughter had the courage to say she had the capacity to be a guest on a podcast. She had the courage to show up to her own life. It was a powerful moment for me, seeing my daughter recognize her worth at such a young age.

Releasing my podcast was super scary for me. Writing this book was super scary for me. Yet, I was amazed to see my daughter have the confidence and courage I truly didn't have when I was her age. As my mission in the world expanded to two businesses and more team members, I was committed to leading with Emotional Intelligence. I was all-in on showing up with the same level of courage and integrity in every aspect of my life. The fear of not being good enough, not being deserving and that people would figure it out and abandon me followed me everywhere. It was so pervasive, and we each have a different way of telling ourselves this narrative. The track in my brain was that I had slipped through the cracks. That I had somehow fooled my husband to think I was worthy of marriage and sooner or later my daughter would realize I wasn't cut out to be a mom. Working through my own stuff, my negative core beliefs about my relationships, the tension, the fighting, the disbelief I could thrive, has really led me to where I am today. I needed to work through these beliefs, and not just in my head, but through practice, and in all of my relationships, especially the ones with my husband, my daughter, and my mother. I had started my podcast to break the silence in my family, and the fact that my daughter and I were having this discussion and she wanted to talk publicly about how I stressed her out as a parent went against everything I ever believed growing up, and I am totally here for it. Growing up, I was very risk averse. In fact, for me to become an entrepreneur was a huge overhaul in my thinking. My daughter, on the other hand, is very much interested in entrepreneurship, which is a term she had heard from me last Thanksgiving. My in-laws came over, we were sitting in our dining room, and we had these great napkins from Urban Barn with conversation starters on them. My conversation starter was,

"Tell us what is the best decision you have ever made," and I had two responses. One was marrying my husband, and the second was becoming an entrepreneur because both allowed me to become the fullness of who I am. Soon after that, my daughter asked me what an entrepreneur was, and we talked about all the trials, tribulations, creativity, growth and personal expansion that came with it. Now, she tells me she really wants to be an entrepreneur, and it just shows me how much, as parents, we really do lead by example.

When I think of her mindset, it's so much more evolved than mine was at her age, and I just love that she has the courage to see herself in this way. This is what I want for the women that I work with. This is what I want for you. I want to help you transform your relationships so that you can fully contribute to your mission. Even though I had limiting beliefs, there was still this fire inside of me that told me my life was meant for more. I knew to some degree that part of my mission was to teach through modeling, transparency and mentorship, and I knew the biggest thing in my way was that I didn't feel confident in my ability to navigate my relationships and my emotions. I had felt like I was one person professionally and a completely different person at home. I felt like a person who wasn't confident, speaking her truth, assertive or asking for her needs to be met. I knew that in order for me to dial into my mission, I needed to master my emotions, learn to communicate fearlessly, and show up in a way that would elevate my relationships.

TRUST ME. YOU GOT THIS.

Remember my commitment to you in the beginning of this book? *I, Dr. Shyamala Kiru, solemnly swear that I will provide you a proven framework that guides you in your journey of becoming an Emotionally Intelligent Woman, offer you strategies to recognize where your own mindset may be holding you back and how to shift to master your emotions, lead with confidence, and communicate fearlessly in all of your relationships, which, in turn, will help you achieve those bigger-than-life dreams I know you have.*

And I will help you adjust your Emotionally Intelligent crown so that you can stand tall like the queen I know you are. Well, now it's time for you to commit to yourself.

You have learned about thinking traps. you have started to dig a little deeper and look at some core beliefs that might have been getting you stuck, and you have begun to develop some high-powered beliefs that will show you **how to get a handle on your emotions.** Remember those pesky thinking traps? How can you forget, right? You learned about anxiety provokers, confidence killers, relationship toxins and Communication Culprits. You learned, not just **how to communicate fearlessly,** but exactly what that sounds like, in practice. That means tossing aside all those unhelpful tactics and understanding how to be assertive and direct. You learned **how to develop a secure attachment style** so you can build those **elevated relationships** and **lead with confidence,** and now, it's time to step into the life you want to live.

DESIGN YOUR BLUEPRINT

I have given you the tools, but the ultimate transformation is in your hands. Now, it's up to YOU to use those tools and design your own blueprint. The one you were always meant for, the one you deserve and is rightfully yours. Take all the learnings, even my own missteps from my life I shared with you, and implement them into your life, remembering the actionable frameworks to get you out of your own way. Get out your pen and notebook, and write down one core concept that you are going to master in the next few weeks. Maybe you start at the beginning of this book and work your way through or jump into a concept that you really feel you need at this time. Commit to doing that over the next week, and the week after, and the next month. You see where I am going with this? The work is lifelong. So, remember, "It's not a sprint, it's a marathon."

I want you to also note that the change you are making isn't for anyone, but you. My husband isn't a man of many words. In fact, my love language is words of affirmation while his is acts of service. Now, something to know about me is that I say "I love you" for everything. That is just who I am, and the other day, my husband texted me saying, "I am going to go return something at Golf Town," to which I replied, "Ok, love you" with heart emojis. After that, he just sent me a text saying, "Okay, then clean the shower," and that was the end of the conversation. I actually posted a screenshot of this conversation on social media and I was so surprised when so many women asked how I had handled that conversation. The truth is that it wasn't a problem for me, and this is something I really want you to consider. It's possible that you will not get verbal affirmation for the changes you are making in your life. I knew my husband wasn't going to be the type to say, "Oh, honey, I see such a difference in you," and the thing is, your partner might be the same way. There are some people who do communicate in that way, but my partner is definitely not one of them, and many of the partners of the women I work with don't either. Sometimes, we look for that external validation of our progress, but it is important to remember you are making these changes for you, not anyone else. You have to validate your own progress.

Back in the day, that text conversation would have really bothered me if my husband had not responded with "I love you, too," but there is truth to the message he did send. His love language is acts of service, and he feels very loved and cared for when I clean the shower. He sees that as a true expression of love. So, I don't feel offended. Instead, I feel secure in how I show up and in our relationship, whether he says I love you or not. Now, whether others validate or even notice your progress or not, don't let it impact your mood. You do not get to choose how others will show up nor do you want to coerce your partner or loved ones to comment on your changes. Instead, you must remember that you are doing this for you, and you are the only person who is really going to see and understand and be proud of the progress you are making. If anything, I want you to know that I am proud of you. I see and validate your progress.

I BELIEVE IN YOU BECAUSE I AM YOU

I am on the exact same journey as you are, and I still do this work every damn day. I see you. You are a high achiever, and you are very good at what you do. I see you climbing that ladder and reaching heights in your career. I see you already wearing your Emotionally Intelligent crown, and sometimes, life may cause it to tilt a little, but I know you can readjust, straighten it, and stand tall. Remind yourself of your mission and remember your inner work. Do not listen to the woman you once were, but listen to the woman you are becoming. Don't forget how far you have come. You have everything you need to succeed both personally and professionally, and there may be bumps and setbacks along the way, but the goal is to keep moving forward. You got this. You *are* an Emotionally Intelligent Woman who is mastering her emotions, communicating fearlessly, and elevating her relationships. You showed up ready, you stayed the course, and now, you are on your way. I am on the exact same journey as you are, and I still do this work every damn day. I see you. You are a high achiever, and you are very good at what you do. I see you climbing that ladder and reaching new heights in your career. I see you already wearing your Emotionally Intelligent crown, and sometimes, life may cause it to tilt a little, but I know you can readjust, straighten it, and stand tall. Remind yourself of your mission and remember your inner work. Do not listen to the woman you once were, but listen to the woman you are becoming. Don't forget how far you have come. You have everything you need to succeed both personally and professionally, and there may be bumps and setbacks along the way, but the goal is to keep moving forward. You got this. You are an Emotionally Intelligent Woman who is mastering her emotions, communicating fearlessly, elevating her relationships and leading with confidence. You showed up ready, you stayed the course, and now, you are on your way. Stand up tall and know that you have someone who believes in you.

DEAR READER

So, here we are. At the end of one journey together, and, perhaps, at the beginning of another. For me, personal growth and expansion over a lifetime is my chosen paradigm of change. Transformation occurs not in a linear fashion, but in an ever expanding, circular fashion. My journey of transformation was never easy. It was never linear, and it wasn't always clear where I would land along the way. What I do know is that, when we approach the process of transformation with courage and integrity, we open ourselves up to living life more fully, more authentically and with more meaning.

Somewhere along the way, I made a decision. I resolved that I would no longer take the easy road, but instead, take the road less traveled. For many women, the idea of taking radical responsibility for our realities and our results, communicating our needs without reservation and showing up powerfully in our relationships is, truly, the road less traveled. For many of us, we may not have had a mother, mentor or guide to show us the path of **Emotional Mastery**, **Fearless Communication**, or to **Lead with Confidence**. For many of us, we may not have ever had someone remind us that we are powerful beyond measure and that our voice is absolutely needed in this world. And, for many of us, we may not have had a community of like-minded women who have also made this decision: to live life on their own terms and to expand fully.

As we walk our final leg of this journey together, what have you decided? What have you resolved in your heart, soul and mind? Who do you want to BECOME in this lifetime? What is your mission

in this world? And finally, who needs you to show up as the most beautiful, radiant and powerful version of yourself?

I believe that it takes a village to raise a fierce woman. I would be nowhere close to my own personal growth and expansion if it had not been for my mentors, guides and teachers. I would be nowhere close to my own mission if it had not been for a community of Emotionally Intelligent Women to hold me accountable to the calling in my heart. If you are feeling nervous, afraid or overwhelmed, please know that you are not alone. The Emotionally Intelligent Woman is a movement that is supportive, expansive and deeply enriching. If you'd like to join us, we'd love to have you. Personal growth and expansion over a lifetime awaits.

With all my love,
Dr. Shyamala

ACKNOWLEDGMENTS

Writing this book has not only been a dream of mine for well over a decade, but it has also been one of the most transformative experiences of my life. While my name may appear as the author, none of this would have been possible without the following individuals.

To my incredible team at Life to Paper Publishing, you walked so closely with me, captured my vision and clarified my teachings. Flor, thank you for your dedication to this work—you served with such passion. Tabitha, thank you for your heart—you are a rare and beautiful soul.

To my very first mentor, Marion, thank you. I will never forget our conversations at the Second Cup. More than the words spoken, your presence and energy were my first encounter with the Emotionally Intelligent Woman. You lead by example, and I am grateful for your contributions to my life and my work.

To my clients, what a sacred journey we've traveled together. Every tear, every story, every milestone continues to live within me. Your resilience, your resolve and your desire for more has always been my reward. Thank you for allowing me to walk with you.

To my parents, where do I even begin? You believed in me with such intensity it scared me at times. Immigrating to Canada with $200 in your pocket, you managed to give me every opportunity in the world. None of what I do and who I am would be possible without your love. Thank you, Mom and Dad. I am eternally grateful for every last bit of who you are.

To my husband, I've never met anyone who could push me so far out of my comfort zone and hold me in such safety, all at the same time. You are more than I could have ever asked for or imagined. You've been waiting for me to write this book for a very long time. Thank you for standing by me as I became the woman who could tell this story.

Finally, to my daughter, if it wasn't for you, the teachings, concepts and ideas inside this book would have never been birthed. Becoming the woman who is called to be your mom is the greatest joy of my life. Thank you for igniting in me the desire to be the best version of myself, and to create the framework for The Emotionally Intelligent Woman.

BIBLIOGRAPHY

1. Ainsworth, Mary. *Patterns of Attachment: A Psychological Study of the Strange Situation.* Psychology Press. 1979.

2. Bowlby, John. *Maternal Deprivation Theory.* 1958.

3. Fleming, Victor. *The Wizard of Oz.* Metro-Goldwyn-Mayer. 1939.

4. Gottman, John. *The Four Horsemen: Criticism, Contempt, Defensiveness, and Stonewalling.* The Gottman Institute. 2013.

5. Howard, Ron. *How the Grinch Stole Christmas.* Imagine Entertainment. 2000.

6. Johnson, Susan (Sue) M. *Attachment Theory in Practice.* The Guilford Press. 2019.

7. Kabat-Zinn, John. *Full Living Catastrophe (Revised Edition): Using the Wisdom of Your Body and Mind to Face Stress, Pain, and Illness.* Bantam. Random House. 2013.

8. Kiru, Shyamala. *Confessions of an Ex-Therapist.* 2021.

9. Kiru, Shyamala. *Kiru Wellness Clinic.* Ontario, Canada.

10. Murakami, Haruki. *What I Talk About When I Talk About Running.* Vintage. 2009.

11. Oswald, Dan. *The Oswald Letter.* HR Daily Advisor. 2010.

12. Siegel, Dan. *Mindsight: The New Science of Personal Transformation.* Bantam. Random House. 2010.

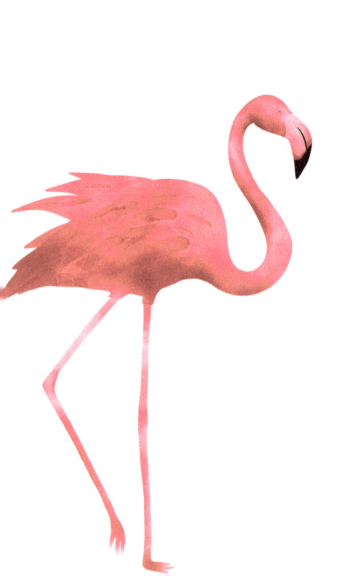

GLOSSARY OF TERMS

1. **Aggressive style** A style of communication marked by a need to maintain control and manipulate others.
2. **Anxious attachment** An attachment style characterized by the intense distress felt when separated from a loved one, which can lead to feelings of sadness, intense loneliness and anxiety.
3. **Assertive style** A style of communication that focuses on maintaining respect for others as well as respect for ourselves and expressing ourselves and our needs, feelings and ideas directly without feeling the need to be right at all times.
4. **Avoidant attachment** An attachment style characterized by the lack of distress felt when separated from a loved one, which can lead to feelings of sadness and loneliness because you are constantly pulling away and creating too much space in your relationships.
5. **Boundaries** Where we draw a line in our relationships to balance the relationships.
6. **Catastrophizing** A thinking trap that occurs when we remove ourselves from reality and place ourselves in a fear zone of catastrophic thoughts.

7. **Communication Culprits** The things done wrong in communication, which can include being passive, aggressive or passive aggressive, failing to communicate at all, and demanding something of someone without taking into account their own needs and wants.

8. **Contempt** A toxic relationship habit and intense expression of criticism where we feel disgust towards another person, making it virtually impossible to resolve conflict.

9. **Core beliefs** Beliefs that are long standing and enduring about ourselves, people and the world; what we tell ourselves despite any evidence that may contradict them.

10. **Criticism** A toxic relationship habit where we make another person feel bad about who they are and what their wants and needs are.

11. **Defensiveness** A toxic relationship habit where we respond defensively in the face of criticism or contempt.

12. **Differentiation** What allows us to balance our individuality and connection in relationships.

13. **Elevated Relationships** Relationships built with secure connections and confidence that allow for feedback and where each person in the relationship is responsible for their own emotions and communication style.

14. **Emotional Intelligence** The capacity to be aware of, in control of, and express our emotions while handling feedback, decision-making, communicating and holding space.

15. **Emotional Mastery** The ability to be aware of and to regulate our emotions in order to take complete responsibility for our own happiness. The ability to feel calm and confident, regardless of external circumstances.

16. **Emotional reasoning** Thoughts we have to ourselves that have no evidence to back it up and can lead to havoc in relationships and mental states because we believe the feeling or emotion to be true despite the fact it is not.

17. **Fearless Communication** The ability to have difficult conversations and ask for what we need, regardless of the outcome.
18. **High-level differentiation** Communicating fearlessly, self-soothing our own anxieties where we can meet the needs of our loved ones and allow ourselves to show up as our best selves in all of our relationships.
19. **High-powered beliefs** Core beliefs that allow us to live our lives fully through flexible thinking and understanding that we are all equals.
20. **Labeling** A thinking trap that occurs when we repeatedly tell ourselves negative labels about ourselves and/or others.
21. **Limiting core beliefs** Core beliefs that hurt our growth and hold us back from becoming Emotionally Intelligent Women.
22. **Low-level differentiation** Losing our sense of self and individuality in a relationship where it is not okay to be direct, open or honest.
23. **Mindfulness** Defined by Jon Kabat-Zinn, mindfulness is "the awareness that arises through paying attention, on purpose, in the present moment, non-judgmentally."
24. **Mind reading** A protective strategy we subconsciously use to keep ourselves safe from criticism that creates social anxiety and places us in constant worry about what others think about us, leaving us unable to authentically express ourselves.
25. **Passive aggressive style** A style of communication marked by the need to want everything to go our way without taking responsibility for our actions or needs.
26. **Passive style** A style of communication marked by the avoidance of conflict, which leads to resentment and strained relationships.

27. **Perfectionism** A thinking trap where there is no room for failure, a need for control and we expect too much of ourselves, setting us up for disappointment.
28. **Personalizing** A thinking trap prompted by fear, a particular sensitivity towards rejection, fueled by self-blame that makes us think that everything is about us, and everything is a negative reflection of us.
29. **Primary emotions** The emotions we carry deep inside us and have suppressed deep down that triggers us.
30. **Proximity maintenance** An element of attachment where we desire to be close to loved ones and maintain physical closeness.
31. **Safe haven** An element of attachment where we continue the process of independence while beginning to tolerate separateness.
32. **Secondary emotions** The emotions we can see and openly express that we are most familiar with.
33. **Secure attachment** An attachment style characterized by the ability to be close and trusting of others while simultaneously feeling empowered towards independence and separateness.
34. **Secure base** An element of attachment where we feel securely and safely attached and have the courage to take more risks and step out of our comfort zones.
35. **Separateness** Recognizing "I am me and you are you" in relationships where there is tolerance for being apart.
36. **Separation distress** An element of attachment where we have difficulty saying goodbye to a loved one and express anxiety or distress during the separation.
37. **Thinking traps** When we operate out of a fear-based reality and consist of catastrophizing, labeling, personalizing and perfectionism.

38. **Togetherness** Emotional and physical closeness that can lead to connection.

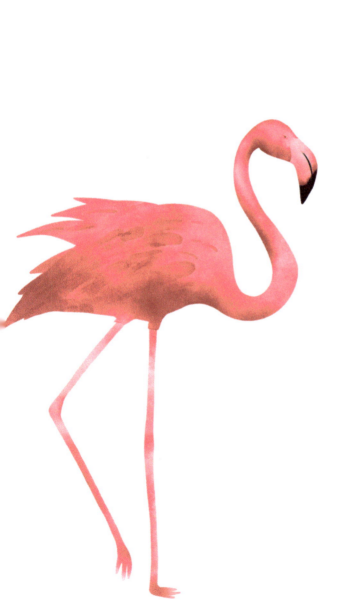

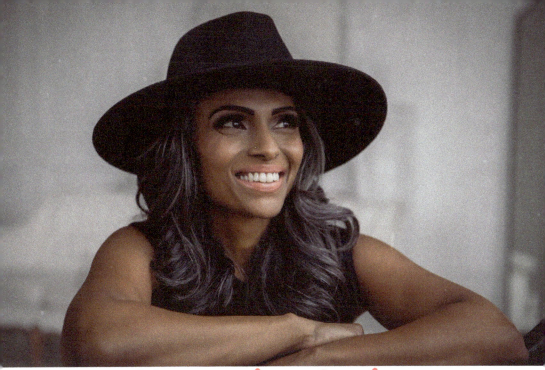

About The Author

Dr. Shyamala is an ex-therapist turned Leadership + Relationship Expert with 20 years experience in advanced communication, relationship management and leadership training for high-powered women.

She is the founder of The EQ Code, a global coaching company designed for women who are ready to master their emotions, communicate fearlessly and lead with confidence, so they can execute on their mission at a whole new level.

While she no longer practices Psychotherapy, she is the founder of the Kiru Psychotherapy Clinic, a virtual mental health practice serving Canada, and has served on the Board of Directors for the Ontario Association for Marriage & Family Therapy.

As a speaker, Dr. Shyamala provides keynote speeches on a local, national and international scale. As a media expert, she's appeared on a national television show for nearly a decade and makes guest appearances on CTV, CP24 as well as frequent pieces of print media.

You can also catch her wisdom on her podcast, Confessions of an Ex-Therapist.

Most importantly, she is the Partner in Crime to her adored husband and the Chief Inspiring Officer to her incredible daughter.

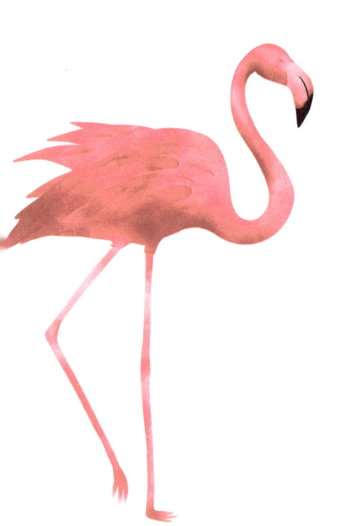

ABOUT THE EQ CODE

The EQ Code is a global coaching company dedicated to helping professional women and female entrepreneurs leverage Emotional Intelligence to increase their capacity for success, both personally and professionally.

Based on our unique methodology, participants are taken through a transformational step-by-step process that allows them to master their emotions, communicate fearlessly and lead with confidence, so they can execute on their mission at a whole new level.

By the end of the program, women report the following 4 outcomes:

1. The ability to feel calm and confident, regardless of external circumstances.
2. The ability to ask for what they need, regardless of how difficult the conversation might be.
3. The ability to navigate their relationships and set boundaries without guilt.
4. The ability to lead themselves and their mission, with complete confidence.

To learn more about joining a global movement of women who are committed to BECOMING the most Emotionally Intelligent version of themselves, check out The EQ Code: www.theeqcode.com

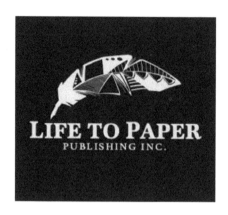

Life to Paper Publishing Inc. (Life to Paper) is an independent publishing house, which helps diverse, mission-driven, heart-centred individuals put their life to paper and reach and inspire audiences and readers.

Life to Paper takes a unique approach to publishing, providing not only ghostwriting, editing and hybrid-publishing services, but also marketing, branding and public relations services, to help individuals take their story from "book I wrote once" to bestseller.

Thanks to our team and partners, we are able to distribute books worldwide that touch the lives and hearts of readers. We guide our authors to discover their unique gifts and empower them to start delivering these talents to the world; therefore, achieving their dream come true and beyond.

Life to Paper aims to allow others to see an author's deepest truths that guide them on a journey to stare directly into their own. We foster storytellers because we believe that "your story can be someone's spark", and change a life.

The Bookshop by Life to Paper is a physical bookstore, which serves the community of Buena Vista, Miami, Florida. We decided to open our doors even further, supporting local authors and artists and providing a place for future authors to commence working on their stories and workshop their pieces through our literary society. The Bookshop by Life to Paper is a place of inspiration and community, showcasing that, if you set your mind to it, you can write the book of your dreams, and we'll help you along the way.

Life to Legacy Foundation is Life to Paper Publishing's not-for-profit organization dedicated to educating and empowering individuals with courses, books and resources to write their life stories. We believe we can change the world one story at a time, and the Life to Legacy Foundation is our way of giving back to all the communities that deserve to have their stories shared.

CPSIA information can be obtained
at www.ICGtesting.com
Printed in the USA
LVHW071951210222
711654LV00023B/412/J

9 781777 373627